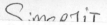

MW01016219

# WORKBOOK TO ACCOMPANY

# Homemaker/Home Health Aide

## FIFTH EDITION

### Mary E. Rizzuto, MSN, RN, CS, CNAA

Administrator, Allied Primary Home Care, San Antonio, Texas

Owner, Team Home Care, Houston, Texas

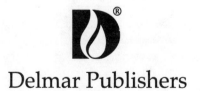

## Delmar Publishers

*an International Thomson Publishing company* I**T**P®

Albany • Bonn • Boston • Cincinnati • Detroit • London • Madrid
Melbourne • Mexico City • New York • Pacific Grove • Paris • San Francisco
Singapore • Tokyo • Toronto • Washington

**NOTICE TO THE READER**

COPYRIGHT © 1998
Delmar is a division of Thomson Learning. The Thomson Learning logo is a registered trademark used herein under license.

Printed in the United States of America
2 3 4 5 6 7 8 9 10 XXX 02 01 00

For more information, contact Delmar, 3 Columbia Circle, PO Box 15015, Albany, NY 12212-0515; or find us on the World Wide Web at http://www.delmar.com

**International Division List**

**Japan:**
Thomson Learning
Palaceside Building 5F
1-1-1 Hitotsubashi, Chiyoda-ku
Tokyo 100 0003 Japan
Tel: 813 5218 6544
Fax: 813 5218 6551

**Australia/New Zealand**
Nelson/Thomson Learning
102 Dodds Street
South Melbourne, Victoria 3205
Australia
Tel: 61 39 685 4111
Fax: 61 39 685 4199

**UK/Europe/Middle East:**
Thomson Learning
Berkshire House
168-173 High Holborn
London
WC1V 7AA United Kingdom
Tel: 44 171 497 1422
Fax: 44 171 497 1426

**Latin America:**
Thomson Learning
Seneca, 53
Colonia Polanco
11560 Mexico D.F. Mexico
Tel: 525-281-2906
Fax: 525-281-2656

**Canada:**
Nelson/Thomson Learning
1120 Birchmount Road
Scarborough, Ontario
Canada M1K 5G4
Tel: 416-752-9100
Fax: 416-752-8102

**Asia:**
Thomson Learning
60 Albert Street, #15-01
Albert Complex
Singapore 189969
Tel: 65 336 6411
Fax: 65 336 7411

ISBN: 0-8273-8086-0

**Library of Congress Catalog Card Number:** 97-12232

# Contents

## INTRODUCTION TO THE STUDENT ············

This workbook was written to assist you in your studies to become part of the home care team as a home health aide. You will use it as you learn about your chosen career. The workbook is divided into five sections.

Section 1 includes the objectives for each chapter in the text and the key terms you will need to learn.

Section 2 includes many application exercises to apply what you have learned.

Section 3 includes crossword puzzles to give you practice in learning vocabulary.

Section 4 includes quizzes to test your knowledge of the material in each unit.

Section 5 includes case studies that will give you an opportunity to apply what you have learned. Every effort has been made to make these case studies realistic.

As you develop your skills and knowledge to become a member of the health care team, you will be working under a supervisor. This supervisor could be a nurse or other educator. The term *supervisor* is meant to include your direct supervisor, the person to whom you report and are supervised by. Where the term *case manager* appears, the registered nurse in charge of the client is the person being referred to.

# Learning Objectives from Text and Terms to Define

# Unit 1   Home Health Services

## LEARNING OBJECTIVES

*After studying this unit, you should be able to:*

- Name three reasons why the trend toward home care has returned.
- Name two services provided by the home health care aide.
- Name members of the health care team.

- Name a type of health care agency.
- Give an example of a managed care organization.
- Describe a hospice.
- Define cultural diversity.

## TERMS TO DEFINE

1. acute illness _a change from normal body functioning, pathological requiring immediate care._

2. case manager _member of the health care team, who coordinates all the services the client may require in the home._

3. chronic illness _a long-term condition._

4. companion _a person hired to keep a client company or maintain safety._

5. culture _The behaviour patterns arts, beliefs, institutions and all other products of human work._

6. developmentally disabled _a mental or physical impairment, usually apparent at birth and require lifelong or extended care._

7. diversity _The quality of being diverse, different, referring to variety having many shapes and forms._

8. home care aid _Caregiver who works with a client with the goal of assisting the client with independently living under supervision._

9. home health aide _nursing care skills, such as bathing the client, under supervision of a Reg Nurse._

10. home health care agencies _Some of which are hospital affilited that focus on providing medical aspects of care in the home._

11. homemaker _person who performs household duties such as laundry and cooking._

12. homemaker/home health aide _person who assists with general household tasks, personal care and simple nursing duties as feeding and bathing._

13. homemaker/home care agencies _provide a variety of nonmedical home support services._

14. hospice _services are becoming more available to help a terminally ill patient die with dignity._

15. licensed nurse agencies _Home Health agencies that provide private-duty registered nurse licensed practical nurse and skilled therapists._

16. licensed practical nurse (LPN) _provides direct care to client may supervise home care workers._

17. managed care _a method of health care delivery that attempts to cut costs by controlling access to and use of physicians, hospitals, nursing facilities and other forms of care._

18. Medicaid _federally and state-funded program that pays medical costs for those whose income is below a certain level._

19. Medicare _federal program that assists persons over 65 years of age with hospital and medical costs._

20. Omnibus Budget Reconciliation Act (OBRA) _Law that regulates that education and certification of home health aides, work in home health agencies and certified hospices._

21. occupational therapist _a skilled professional who evaluates a clients ability to perform skill necessary to independent living as bathing dressing cooking and the who works with clients to improve these ability_

22. personal care worker _person who assists with minimual level of daily living activities such as companionship and meal preparation._

23. physical therapist _a skilled professional who evaluates a clients ability to stand walk climb stairs transfer and do other activities_

24. physician (MD) _____

25. registered nurse (RN) _____

26. social service agencies _____

27. social worker _____

28. speech therapist _____

29. terminal illness _____

# Unit 2  Responsibilities of the Home Health Aide

## LEARNING OBJECTIVES

*After studying this unit, you should be able to:*

- List three important qualities of the home health aide.
- Give five examples of actions to avoid that can lead to liability.
- Explain why accurate observation, reporting, and documentation are important tasks.
- Give examples of good personal hygiene.
- Define ethics, and identify two examples of ethical practice.
- List five "rights" of the client.
- List three "rights" of the home health aide.
- Define client abuse.
- List four kinds of abuse.

## TERMS TO DEFINE

1. abuse _____

2. career _____

3. components _____

4. confidentiality _____

5. documentation _____

6. ethics _____

7. evaluation _____

8. flexible _____

9. hygiene _____

10. interaction _____

11. interpersonal relationships _____

12. liability _____

13. negligence _____

14. observation _____

15. oral hygiene _____

16. practice _____

17. procedure _____

18. reporting _____

19. theory _____

20. time organization _____

# Unit 3   Developing Effective Communication Skills

## LEARNING OBJECTIVES

*After studying this unit, you should be able to:*

- Explain the difference between verbal and nonverbal communication.
- Define the components of basic communication.
- List factors that promote good communication between worker and supervisor.
- Practice active listening.
- Use some of the techniques to improve communication with clients.
- Be more deliberate in communicating with friends, coworkers, and clients.
- Demonstrate the following:
  Procedure 1   Inserting a Hearing Aid

## TERMS TO DEFINE

1. active listening _____

2. body language _____

3. communication _____

4. invalidate _____

5. listening _____

6. nonverbal communication _____

7. nonjudgmental _____

8. paraphrase _____

9. passive listening _____

10. platitude _____

11. restate _____

# Unit 4  Safety

## LEARNING OBJECTIVES

*After studying this unit, you should be able to:*

- Identify the conditions in aging that contribute to the incidence of accidents.
- Identify five causes of accidents around the home.
- List three assistive safety devices used with the frail elderly.
- State the basic rules to follow in the event of a home fire.
- List five safety tips for the home.
- List 10 rules of good body mechanics.

## TERMS TO DEFINE

1. body mechanics _____

2. evacuate _____

3. fire extinguishers _____

4. gait belt _____

5. hazard _____

6. peripheral vision _____

7. pivot _____

8. synchronize _____

9. transfer belt _____

# Unit 5  Homemaking Service

## LEARNING OBJECTIVES

*After studying this unit, you should be able to:*

- List at least four tips used to plan and organize tasks.
- Explain how to care for major home appliances.
- State some ways to combine client care and household tasks.
- Name three factors that determine the home health aide's cleaning plan.
- List five cleaning tasks done daily.
- List five cleaning tasks done only periodically.
- Describe the correct method for separating and disposing of garbage.
- Identify at least four steps used in cleaning a kitchen.
- Identify bathroom tasks the home health aide does daily.
- List four guidelines for planning menus.
- State eight guidelines for buying food.
- List four guidelines for storing food.
- Name five guidelines for preparing meals.
- Identify two ways to sort clothes for washing.
- Identify several methods for removing stains.
- Explain how to wash the clothing and bed linens of a client with an infectious disease.
- Demonstrate the following:
  Procedure 2   Changing an Unoccupied Bed

## Terms to Define ··················································································

1. bulk _____

2. convenience foods _____

3. delicatessen _____

4. fermented _____

5. Meals on Wheels _____

6. mildew _____

7. pathogens _____

8. perishable _____

9. permanent press _____

10. polyester fabrics _____

11. produce _____

12. recyclable _____

13. sanitary _____

14. staple items _____

# Unit 6    Infancy to Adolescence

## LEARNING OBJECTIVES
··························································

*After studying this unit, you should be able to:*

- Name the five basic human needs.
- Identify three immunizations necessary for infants.
- List six disorders of the newborn.
- List four behavioral patterns associated with abused children.
- Know where and how to report cases of suspected child abuse.

- List four conditions that can occur in an infant if the mother drinks alcohol during pregnancy.
- Describe three characteristics of toddlers.
- Identify three developmental tasks of a preschool-aged child.
- Name two health problems that may affect adolescents.
- Identify changes that occur at puberty.

## Terms to Define ··················································································

1. adolescence _____

2. bonding _____

3. cerebral palsy _____

4. cesarean section _____

5. child abuse _____

6. conception _____

7. cystic fibrosis _____

8. fetal alcohol syndrome _____

9. fetus _____

10. gestation period _____

11. immunity _____

12. low birthweight _____

13. premature _____

14. puberty _____

15. sexually transmitted disease (STD) _____

16. sibling rivalry _____

17. sudden infant death syndrome _____

# Unit 7    Early and Middle Adulthood

## LEARNING OBJECTIVES

*After studying this unit, you should be able to:*

- List the causes of health problems in the early adult years.
- Describe the adjustments that often must be dealt with in the middle adult years.
- State why preventive health measures are important.

- Describe the changes that occur during the early and middle adult years in terms of family relationships.
- List two reasons a home health aide should encourage the client to exercise.
- List two activities a disabled client can become involved in outside of the home.

## TERMS TO DEFINE

1. early adulthood _____

2. empty nest syndrome _____

3. mammogram _____

4. menopause _____

5. middle adulthood _____

6. multiple sclerosis _____

7. Pap smear _____

8. preventive health measure _____

9. prognosis _____

10. rheumatoid arthritis _____

11. self-esteem _____

12. sigmoidoscopy _____

# Unit 8   Older Adulthood

## LEARNING OBJECTIVES

*After studying this unit, you should be able to:*

- Name some of the normal age-related changes.
- Describe common changes to hearing and how to help older clients cope.
- Describe common changes to vision and how to help the older person.
- Describe reminiscence and how it can be helpful to an older person with depression or dementia.
- Describe dementia.
- Describe depression.

## TERMS TO DEFINE

1. acuity _____

2. aged _____

3. carbohydrates _____

4. cataracts _____

5. dementia _____

6. depression _____

7. glaucoma _____

8. incontinence _____

9. osteoporosis _____

10. over the counter _____

11. reminiscence _____

12. somaticize _____

# Unit 9   Principles of Infection Control

## LEARNING OBJECTIVES

*After studying this unit, you should be able to:*

- Name three different types of microorganisms.
- Describe standard precautions.
- List three modes of transmission (the ways germs can spread from one person to another).
- List two contagious/infectious diseases.
- Explain signs and symptoms and nursing care for a client with tuberculosis.
- List six rules to follow when caring for a client with an infectious disease.
- Give examples of situations requiring standard precautions.

- Name the single most effective precaution to prevent the spread of infections.
- List five examples of when aides must wash their hands.
- Explain the purpose of each procedure.
- Demonstrate the following:
  Procedure 3   Handwashing
  Procedure 4   Gloving
  Procedure 5   Putting on and Removing Personal Protective Equipment
  Procedure 6   Collecting Specimen from Client on Transmission-Based Precautions

## TERMS TO DEFINE

1. aseptic techniques _____
2. bacteria _____
3. contaminated _____
4. disinfected _____
5. fungi _____
6. germs _____
7. hepatitis B _____
8. incubation period _____
9. infection _____
10. infection control _____
11. infectious disease _____
12. isolation _____
13. jaundice _____
14. microorganisms _____
15. pathogens _____
16. protozoa _____

17. rickettsiae _____

18. standard precautions _____

19. sterile _____

20. tuberculosis _____

21. virus _____

# Unit 10  From Wellness to Illness

## LEARNING OBJECTIVES

*After studying this unit, you should be able to:*

- Identify the four vital signs and their normal values.
- Name three body sites where temperature is taken.
- Identify four signs that a client may be ill.
- Define disability.
- Define rehabilitation.
- Describe your role in rehabilitation.
- Describe the care given to an unconscious client.
- Demonstrate the following:
  Procedure  7    Taking an Oral Temperature
  Procedure  8    Taking a Rectal Temperature

Procedure  9    Taking an Axillary Temperature
Procedure 10    Taking a Radial and Apical Pulse
Procedure 11    Counting Respirations
Procedure 12    Taking Blood Pressure
Procedure 13    Measuring Height and Weight
Procedure 14    Assisting the Client with Self-Administered Medications
Procedure 15    Performing Passive Range of Motion Exercises
Procedure 16    Assisting the Client to Walk with Crutches, Walker, or Cane

## TERMS TO DEFINE

1. activities _____

2. acute _____

3. apnea _____

4. blood pressure _____

5. bradycardia _____

6. Cheyne-Stokes _____

7. chronic _____

8. contracture _____

9. diastolic _____

10. disability _____

11. dyspnea _____

12. pulse _____

13. rales _____

14. range of motion exercises _____

15. rehabilitation _____

16. respiration _____

17. sign _____

18. sphygmomanometer _____

19. symptom _____

20. systolic _____

21. tachycardia _____

22. vital signs _____

# Unit 11   Mental Health

## LEARNING OBJECTIVES

*After studying this unit, you should be able to:*

- Identify several common emotions.
- Identify how a physical response can result from an emotional reaction.
- Define mental illness.
- Define psychology, mental health, and adjustments.
- Differentiate between external and internal stimuli.
- Identify the major symptoms of depression.

## TERMS TO DEFINE

1. adjustment _____

2. delirium _____

3. dementia _____

4. depression _____

5. emotions _____

6. empathy _____

7. external stimulus _____

8. internal stimulus _____

9. mental disorders _____

10. optimist _____

11. pessimist _____

12. psychology _____

13. stress _____

# Unit 12   Digestion and Nutrition

## LEARNING OBJECTIVES

*After studying this unit, you should be able to:*

- List the six food groups on the food guide pyramid.
- Identify the special diets used for at least five medical conditions.
- Name six things to keep in mind when planning and preparing meals.

- Name eight special diets that may be prescribed for your client, and describe the types of foods that are usually permitted for each.
- Identify the special diet a client with acquired immunodeficiency syndrome (AIDS) would require.
- Demonstrate the following:
  Procedure 17   Feeding the Client

## TERMS TO DEFINE

1. bland diet _____

2. calorie-controlled diet _____

3. clear liquid diet _____

4. degenerative diseases _____

5. diabetic diet _____

6. diuretic _____

7. emesis _____

8. empty calorie _____

9. feces _____

10. fiber _____

11. food allergy _____

12. food guide pyramid _____

13. full-liquid diet _____

14. high-fiber diet _____

15. impacted _____

16. low-residue diet _____

17. low-sodium diet _____

18. malnutrition _____

19. Meals on Wheels _____

20. metabolism _____

21. nutrition _____

22. peristalsis _____

23. pureed diet _____

24. soft diet _____

25. stool _____

26. vegetarians _____

# Unit 13   Elimination

## LEARNING OBJECTIVES

*After studying this unit, you should be able to:*

- Identify the structures of male and female urinary tracts.
- Describe three types of urinary incontinence.
- Demonstrate the following:

| | |
|---|---|
| Procedure 18 | Measuring and Recording Fluid Intake and Output |
| Procedure 19 | Giving and Emptying the Bedpan |
| Procedure 20 | Giving and Emptying the Urinal |
| Procedure 21 | Collecting a Clean-Catch Urine Specimen |
| Procedure 22 | Caring for a Urinary Catheter |
| Procedure 23 | Connecting the Leg Bag |
| Procedure 24 | Emptying a Drainage Unit |
| Procedure 25 | Retraining the Bladder |
| Procedure 26 | Giving a Commercial Enema |
| Procedure 27 | Giving a Rectal Suppository |
| Procedure 28 | Retraining the Bowels |
| Procedure 29 | Applying Adult Briefs |
| Procedure 30 | Collecting a Stool Specimen |
| Procedure 31 | Assisting with Changing an Ostomy Bag |

## TERMS TO DEFINE

1. bladder _____

2. clean-catch specimen _____

3. constipation _____

4. cystitis _____

5. detrusor instability _____

6. enema _____

7. impaction _____

8. incontinent _____

9. kidney _____

10. kidney stones _____

11. ostomy bag _____

12. perineum _____

13. stoma _____

14. suppository _____

15. urinary catheter _____

16. ureters _____

17. urethra _____

# Unit 14  Integumentary System

## LEARNING OBJECTIVES

*After studying this unit, you should be able to:*

- Identify one function of the integumentary system.
- List the symptoms of pressure sore development.
- Describe good skin care.
- Describe treatment of heatstroke.
- Demonstrate the following:

| | |
|---|---|
| Procedure 32 | Applying Clean Dressing and Ointment to Broken Skin |
| Procedure 33 | Assisting with Tub Bath or Shower |
| Procedure 34 | Giving a Bed Bath |
| Procedure 35 | Giving a Backrub |
| Procedure 36 | Giving Female Perineal Care |
| Procedure 37 | Giving Male Perineal Care |
| Procedure 38 | Assisting with Routine Oral Hygiene |
| Procedure 39 | Caring for Dentures |
| Procedure 40 | Shaving the Male Client |
| Procedure 41 | Performing a Warm Foot Soak |
| Procedure 42 | Giving Nail Care |
| Procedure 43 | Shampooing the Client's Hair in Bed |
| Procedure 44 | Caring for an Artificial Eye |

## TERMS TO DEFINE

1. bony prominence _____

2. dermis _____

3. epidermis _____

4. hyperthermia _____

5. hypothermia _____

6. perineum _____

7. pressure sores _____

# Unit 15 Musculoskeletal System: Arthritis, Body Mechanics, and Restorative Care

## LEARNING OBJECTIVES

*After studying this unit, you should be able to:*

- Describe the care given to clients with arthritis.
- Define the terms relating to arthritis.
- Discuss the exercises related to arthritis.
- Define osteoarthritis, rheumatoid arthritis, and gout.
- List two types of diets that may be prescribed for clients with arthritis.
- List three side effects of steroids.
- List two goals of an exercise program for a client with arthritis.
- Name two joints that can be replaced by surgery.
- Demonstrate the following:
  Procedure 45  Turning the Client Toward You
  Procedure 46  Moving the Client Up in Bed Using the Drawsheet
  Procedure 47  Making an Occupied Bed
  Procedure 48  Log Rolling the Client
  Procedure 49  Positioning the Client in Supine Position

  Procedure 50  Positioning the Client in Lateral/Side-Lying Position
  Procedure 51  Positioning the Client in Prone Position
  Procedure 52  Positioning the Client in Fowler's Position
  Procedure 53  Assisting the Client from Bed to Wheelchair
  Procedure 54  Assisting the Client from Wheelchair to Bed
  Procedure 55  Transferring the Client from Wheelchair to Toilet/Commode
  Procedure 56  Lifting the Client Using a Mechanical Lift
  Procedure 57  Caring for Casts
  Procedure 58  Applying an Ice Bag, Cap, or Collar
  Procedure 59  Dressing and Undressing the Client

## TERMS TO DEFINE

1. anti-inflammatory _____

2. arthritis _____

3. degenerative disease _____

4. fracture _____

5. gout _____

6. ligaments _____

7. osteoarthritis _____

8. rheumatism _____

9. rheumatoid arthritis _____

10. steroids _____

11. tophi _____

# Unit 16   Nervous System

## LEARNING OBJECTIVES

*After studying this unit, you should be able to:*

- Define paraplegia, quadriplegia, and hemiplegia.
- Identify three common sensory losses in older adults.
- Name and describe four common sensory disorders.

- Describe the following:
  Procedure 60   Caring for a Client Having a Seizure

### TERMS TO DEFINE

1. amyotrophic lateral sclerosis (ALS) _____

2. auditory _____

3. cerebral vascular accident (CVA) _____

4. hemiplegia _____

5. multiple sclerosis (MS) _____

6. muscular dystrophy _____

7. otosclerosis _____

8. paraplegia _____

9. Parkinson's disease _____

10. quadriplegia _____

11. seizure _____

12. sensory deficits _____

# Unit 17   Circulatory System

## LEARNING OBJECTIVES

*After studying this unit, you should be able to:*

- Identify symptoms of four heart conditions.
- Describe care given for clients with heart conditions.

- Explain the effect nitroglycerin has on the blood vessels.
- Give two other names for a CVA.

- List six risk factors for heart attacks and strokes.
- List three signs a client might display if suffering from a heart attack.
- List four warning signs of stroke.
- List three causes of stroke.
- List two types of aphasia.
- List three physical defects a client may have after a stroke.

- Explain the role of the aide in assisting a client recovering from a stroke.
- List three blood disorders.
- List three symptoms of arterial insufficiency.
- Describe three ways the aide can assist in the care of a client with thrombophlebitis.
- Demonstrate the following:
  Procedure 61   Applying Elasticized Stockings

## TERMS TO DEFINE

1. activities of daily living (ADL) _____

2. anemia _____

3. aneurysm _____

4. angina pectoris _____

5. anticoagulants _____

6. aphasia _____

7. arterial insufficiency _____

8. arteriogram _____

9. arteriosclerosis _____

10. artery _____

11. atherosclerosis _____

12. cardiac arrest _____

13. catheterization _____

14. cerebral hemorrhage _____

15. cerebral infarction _____

16. cerebral vascular accident (CVA) _____

17. collateral circulation _____

18. congestive heart failure _____

19. cyanosis _____

20. edema _____

21. embolus _____

22. expressive aphasia _____

23. gangrene _____

24. hemophilia _____

25. hypertension _____

26. hypotension _____

27. intermittent claudication _____

28. ischemia _____

29. leukemia _____

30. multi-infarct dementia _____

31. myocardial infarction _____

32. myocardium _____

33. nitroglycerin _____

34. occupational therapist _____

35. phlebitis _____

36. pulmonary embolus _____

37. receptive aphasia _____

38. sickle cell anemia _____

39. sublingually _____

40. thrombophlebitis _____

41. thrombus _____

42. transient ischemic attack (TIA) _____

43. venous insufficiency _____

# Unit 18   Respiratory System

## LEARNING OBJECTIVES

*After studying this unit, you should be able to:*

- Discuss the basic function of the respiratory system.
- Name the major organs of the respiratory system.
- Define pneumonia, chronic bronchitis, emphysema, and asthma. (Include at least 1 symptom and 1 intervention for each illness.)

- Demonstrate the following:

| Procedure 62 | Collecting a Sputum Specimen |
| Procedure 63 | Assisting with Coughing and Deep-Breathing Exercises |
| Procedure 64 | Assisting the Client with Oxygen Therapy |

## TERMS TO DEFINE ·····················································

1. asthma _____

2. chronic bronchitis _____

3. chronic obstructive pulmonary disease (COPD) _____

4. emphysema _____

5. pneumonia _____

6. respiratory system _____

# Unit 19    Reproductive System

## LEARNING OBJECTIVES
·····················································

*After studying this unit, you should be able to:*

- Identify the male and female reproductive organs.
- Describe the functions of each major organ.
- Name three common disorders of the reproductive system.

- List five sexually transmitted diseases and their symptoms.
- List and describe male and female hormones and their functions.

## TERMS TO DEFINE ·····················································

1. cervix _____

2. dysmenorrhea _____

3. ectopic pregnancy _____

4. estrogen _____

5. fallopian tubes _____

6. genital herpes _____

7. genitalia _____

8. gonorrhea _____

9. gynecologist _____

10. menopause _____

11. menstruation _____

12. nongonococcal urethritis _____

13. ovaries _____

14. pelvic inflammatory disease _____

15. penis _____

16. progesterone _____

17. scrotum _____

18. sexually transmitted disease (STD) _____

19. syphilis _____

20. testes _____

21. testosterone _____

22. urethra _____

23. uterus _____

24. vagina _____

25. vaginitis _____

26. vulva _____

# Unit 20   Endocrine System and Diabetes

## LEARNING OBJECTIVES

*After studying this unit, you should be able to:*

- Name four signs and symptoms of diabetes.
- List four types of diabetes mellitus.
- Name three ways of controlling diabetes.
- Name three long-term complications of diabetes.
- List signs and symptoms for insulin shock and acidosis and the immediate care for each.
- Explain special foot care given to the diabetic client.
- Describe special techniques used in caring for a client who has vision impairment.
- Demonstrate the following:
  Procedure 65   Testing Blood

## TERMS TO DEFINE

1. acidosis _____

2. blood lancet _____

3. cyanotic _____

4. diabetes _____

5. ducts _____

6. endocrine glands _____

7. gangrene _____

8. gestational _____

9. glucometer _____

10. glucose _____

11. hormone _____

12. hyperglycemia _____

13. hyperthyroidism _____

14. hypoglycemia _____

15. hypothyroidism _____

16. insulin _____

17. neuropathy _____

18. subcutaneously _____

# Unit 21   Caring for the Client Who Is Terminally Ill

## LEARNING OBJECTIVES

*After studying this unit, you should be able to:*

- Identify some cultural influences surrounding practices related to death.
- Identify the five stages of dying as described by Dr. Kübler-Ross.
- Identify the home health aide's responsibilities when the client dies.
- Identify ways in which a person may react to the death of a family member or friend.

- Become familiar with the needs of a dying client.
- Explain the Patient Self-Determination Act.
- Explain the purpose of hospice programs.
- Explain the importance of grieving.
- Understand different reactions to dying.

## TERMS TO DEFINE

1. advance directives _____

2. autopsy _____

3. durable power of attorney _____

4. embalming _____

5. grieving _____

6. hospice _____

7. living will _____

8. Patient Self-Determination Act _____

9. terminal _____

# Unit 22   Caring for the Client with Alzheimer's Disease

## LEARNING OBJECTIVES
*After studying this unit, you should be able to:*

- Describe five symptoms of Alzheimer's disease.
- Understand the 10 warning signs of Alzheimer's disease.
- Name at least five interventions to take to promote the safety of a client who wanders.
- Describe several causes of wandering and disruptive behaviors.

- Describe validation therapy, reminiscence, and reality orientation and their value with the Alzheimer's client.
- List 10 tips for communicating with the client who has Alzheimer's disease.

## TERMS TO DEFINE

1. Alzheimer's disease _____

2. dementia _____

3. disruptive behaviors _____

4. reality orientation _____

5. reminiscence _____

6. validation therapy _____

7. wandering _____

# Unit 23   Caring for the Client with Cancer

## LEARNING OBJECTIVES
*After studying this unit, you should be able to:*

- Identify three diagnostic tests for cancer.
- Identify six surgical procedures used in cancer treatment.
- List seven warning signs of cancer.
- Define metastasis, benign tumor, remission, and malignant.

- Name three types of treatment for cancer.
- Describe the care given to a client with cancer.
- List two precautions for an aide to take when caring for a client who is on chemotherapy.
- List side effects commonly demonstrated by clients receiving cancer treatments.

## TERMS TO DEFINE

1. articulates _____

2. benign _____

3. biopsy _____

4. cancer _____

5. carcinogen _____

6. chemotherapy _____

7. colostomy _____

8. expectorate _____

9. hysterectomy _____

10. ileostomy _____

11. irrigation _____

12. laryngectomy _____

13. larynx _____

14. lobectomy _____

15. lumpectomy _____

16. malignant _____

17. mammogram _____

18. mastectomy _____

19. metastasis _____

20. pneumonectomy _____

21. prosthesis _____

22. remission _____

23. stoma _____

24. trachea _____

25. tracheostomy _____

# Unit 24   Caring for the Client with AIDS

## LEARNING OBJECTIVES

*After studying this unit, you should be able to:*

- Understand how HIV is transmitted.
- Understand symptoms of HIV.
- Understand symptom-specific nursing care for clients with HIV.
- Understand necessary precautions to prevent the spread of HIV.

**TERMS TO DEFINE**

1. acquired immunodeficiency syndrome (AIDS) _____

2. human immunodeficiency virus (HIV) _____

3. sexually transmitted disease (STD) _____

# Unit 25   Maternal Care

## LEARNING OBJECTIVES

*After studying this unit, you should be able to:*

- List common pregnancy symptoms and their treatments.
- Identify high-risk pregnancies.
- Recognize danger signals in pregnancy.
- Describe mechanisms for caring for the expectant mother.
- List common postpartum discomforts and their treatments.
- Recognize abnormal postpartum problems.

**TERMS TO DEFINE**

1. breast engorgement _____

2. Down's syndrome _____

3. edema _____

4. engagement _____

5. fetal alcohol syndrome _____

6. flatulence _____

7. heartburn _____

8. hemorrhoids _____

9. high-risk pregnancies _____

10. lochia _____

11. postpartum _____

12. postpartum blues _____

13. varicose veins _____

# Unit 26   Infant Care

## LEARNING OBJECTIVES

*After studying this unit, you should be able to:*

- Understand the proper technique to bottle-feed an infant.
- Identify the procedures for breast-feeding an infant.
- Describe three techniques for burping an infant.
- Decribe the steps to bathe an infant.
- Define circumcision and identify the appropriate care for the circumcised/uncircumcised penis.

- Identify safety precautions to be taken with each infant care procedure.
- Demonstrate the following:
  Procedure 66   Assisting with Breast-Feeding and Breast Care
  Procedure 67   Bottle-Feeding an Infant
  Procedure 68   Burping an Infant
  Procedure 69   Bathing an Infant

## TERMS TO DEFINE

1. bottle-feeding _____

2. breast-feeding _____

3. circumcision _____

4. foreskin _____

5. glans _____

6. lactose _____

# Unit 27   Job-Seeking Skills

## LEARNING OBJECTIVES

*After studying this unit, you should be able to:*

- Identify three trends affecting home health care employment.
- List potential employment sites that hire homemaker/home health aides.
- Prepare a personal information sheet.

- Describe how to present yourself in a professional manner during an employment interview.
- Complete an employment application accurately.
- Give five examples of misconduct on the job.

## TERMS TO DEFINE

1. diagnosis related group system (DRGs) _____

2. information sheet _____

3. infraction _____

4. misconduct _____

5. personal reference _____

6. registry service _____

# SECTION TWO

# Application Exercises

# Unit 1   Home Health Services

## SHORT ANSWER/FILL IN THE BLANKS ···································

Complete the following sentences with the correct word or words.

1. The main purpose of the first homemaker service agency in the United States was to provide _____Child_____ _____Care_____.

2. Home health aides are expected to work under direct supervision of a _____ _____.

3. Minimum training and competency requirements for home health aides were established by the _____ _____ _____ _____, also known as _____.

4. In the earlier years of our country the frail, disabled and elderly were cared for by _____ members.

5. As the country became industrialized, the family unit became smaller, usually consisting of the parents and the children only. This type of family is known as the _____ family.

6. One of the main reasons for the growth of home care is the growth in the _____ _____, the main recipients of home care.

7. _____ cost of hospital care and _____ discharge of patients from hospitals are other reasons for the increase of home care.

8. Many people prefer to remain in their own _____ rather than move to a _____ _____ when they become ill or frail.

9. Home care services for people who prefer to remain at home to die are called _____.

10. Two main categories of duties of home care workers are care of the _____ and care of the _____.

11. Activities of daily living include:

    a. _____

    b. _____

    c. _____

    d. _____

12. Care of the home can include:

    a. _____

    b. _____

    c. _____

    d. _____

13. Each home care client has a separate care plan that is designed by the worker's _____.

14. The home health aide is a member of the health care _____.

15. A federally and state funded program that pays for health care services for persons whose income is below a certain amount is _____.

16. To qualify for Medicare reimbursement for home health, an individual must be:

    a. confined to _____.

    b. under the care of a _____.

    c. in need of _____ _____ _____, _____ _____, or _____ _____.

    d. receiving care from a Medicare _____ _____.

17. Everyone in the United States who has paid into _____ _____ is entitled to apply for Medicare insurance once he or she is _____ years of age or becomes _____.

18. The method of health care delivery that attempts to control costs through the use of gatekeepers controlling access to care is called a _____ _____ _____. They are sometimes referred to as _____.

19. The cost of care to the client is _____ than with traditional insurance; however, the client has less choices of providers.

## MATCHING

Match each term with the proper definition.

20. _____ companion
21. _____ home care aide
22. _____ home health aide
23. _____ personal care worker
24. _____ homemaker/home health aide
25. _____ homemaker

a. assists in general household tasks, as well as those listed for the home health aide

b. performs household duties such as laundry and cooking

c. works with the client with the goal of assisting the client with independent living under professional supervision

d. in the home to keep the client company or to maintain safety, usually does not provide personal or homemaking services

e. assists with a minimal level of daily living activities, such as meal preparation and companionship as well as minimal assistance with personal care

f. able to provide substantial assistance with personal care, such as bathing and dressing

## TRUE OR FALSE

Answer the following statements true (T) or false (F).

26. T   F   The Omnibus Reconciliation Act (OBRA) mandates federal Medicare and Medicaid standards for nursing homes and home health agencies.

27. T   F   A mutual goal of the OBRA, Medicare, and Medicaid regulations is to improve care for individuals in long-term care facilities and for those in their homes.

28. T   F   Medicare is a state program.

29. T  F  The physical therapist authorizes home health care.

30. T  F  Home care clients are diverse and represent many different cultures and ethnic groups.

31. T  F  A chronic illness is one that lasts a short time, requires immediate treatment, and can be expected to go away.

32. T  F  Alzheimer's disease is considered a chronic illness.

33. T  F  Developmentally disabled means a severe chronic disability.

34. T  F  Terminal illnesses are illnesses that individuals are expected to recover from in a short time.

35. T  F  Home health clients come from all ages, all cultures, and all ethnic groups.

36. T  F  Home health aides must be willing to listen to the instructions from their case managers regarding the care of each individual because they cannot expect to know all the different traditions and practices of each client.

37. T  F  A home health aide must instruct the client to follow the religious practices of the home health aide.

38. T  F  A speech therapist assesses the client's ability to stand, walk, and climb stairs.

39. T  F  An occupational therapist evaluates a client's ability to perform activities of daily living.

40. T  F  A social worker gives direct nursing care to the client.

## MULTIPLE CHOICE

Choose the correct answer or answers.

41. Increased need for home care is due to
    a. the increase of HMOs
    b. the shortage of hospital beds
    c. discharge of clients that are sicker and need follow-up care
    d. the shortage of physicians

42. The person who evaluates the client's ability to perform skills necessary to independent living is the
    a. physical therapist
    b. occupational therapist
    c. speech therapist
    d. home health aide

43. A federally and state funded program that pays for health care services for those persons with income below a certain level is called
    a. Medicaid
    b. Medicare
    c. HMOs
    d. food stamps

44. Whenever government funding is involved in health care
    a. there will be much waste
    b. federal regulation of the health care industry will be present
    c. the states will not be involved in regulation
    d. each state will determine its own requirements

45. The person responsible for coordinating the care of the client is
    a. the home health aide
    b. the social worker
    c. the case manager
    d. the office supervisor

## PRACTICE SITUATION ·······································································

46. Joan, a friend of yours, approaches you and tells you she going to have surgery in the next few weeks. Her physician has told her that she will need help in the home after going home. She knows you are becoming a home health aide. She asks you to explain what you do in the home for your clients. She is nervous about having strangers in her home. What information can you give Joan to make her feel more comfortable about care in the home?

_____

_____

47. Refer to Figure 1-1. List six areas the home health aide needs to be aware of in personal appearance.

a. _____

b. _____

c. _____

d. _____

e. _____

f. _____

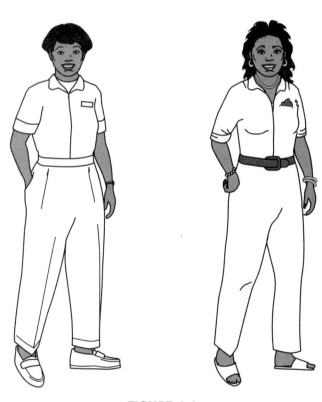

**FIGURE 1-1**

# Unit 2   Responsibilities of the Home Health Aide

## SHORT ANSWER/FILL IN THE BLANKS

Complete the following sentences with the correct word or words.

1. A _____ is the occupation or profession for which one has been specially educated.

2. A home health aide must be flexible, be willing to follow instructions, be _____ organized, have good _____ skills, be _____ _____ _____, and have good personal _____.

3. A home health aide must be able to adjust _____ from one situation to another.

4. The home health aide must treat all clients with _____.

5. The home health aide must be able to _____ to different settings and be able to give _____ and _____ care in each situation.

6. _____ of a job are the separate parts that make up the whole.

7. A _____ is a list of steps used to complete a task.

8. _____ is the information that forms a basis for action.

9. _____ is the actual performance of the procedure.

10. Before assigning a client, the _____ will provide a home care plan for the client, describing the specific duties of the home health aide.

11. The care plan should include duties, client's needs, and the _____ to _____ in case of an emergency.

12. _____ refers to the degree to which you are held responsible for something that goes wrong on the job.

13. The most important _____ from liability is to perform only and exactly what your supervisor instructs you to do.

14. Pitfalls you should avoid in your job include:

    a. doing _____ than is assigned.

    b. doing _____ than is assigned.

    c. doing _____, _____, or poor quality work.

    d. using your car for _____ _____ without notifying your _____ company.

    e. failing to act in an _____.

    f. failing to do accurate reporting and _____.

    g. attempting to do things that are beyond your _____.

h. _____ yourself or your client by doing something you are not assigned or adequately trained to do.

i. failing to report unsafe _____.

15. A home health aide will usually be assigned to more than one client; for the aide to complete the tasks in the proper time frame, the aide will have to be _____.

16. Interactions occur between one or more _____.

17. The home health aide may be the first to notice a _____ with the client.

18. The best way to remove body odors is with _____ and _____.

19. Fingernails should be worn _____ and _____.

20. Dangling necklaces are not worn in the client's home because they may catch on _____.

21. Perfumes are sometimes _____ to clients.

22. If the skin is broken or scratches, there is always danger of _____.

23. _____ is a code or standard of behavior. It is a code concerned with what is _____ and what is _____.

24. Dishonesty not only involves the taking of objects or money, but also means not _____ reports.

25. Home health aides should _____ discuss their clients with anyone except their supervisors.

26. If a client offers you a gift, you should do what?

_____

_____

27. If a client becomes rude, what would you do to handle it?

_____

_____

28. Medicare and Medicaid have mandated a list of rights of clients that must be given to each client that is funded by the government. Five of them are:

a. _____

b. _____

c. _____

d. _____

e. _____

29. Five rights you have as a home health aide are:

   a. _____

   b. _____

   c. _____

   d. _____

   e. _____

30. Client abuse may be:

   a. _____

   b. _____

   c. _____

   d. _____

## TRUE OR FALSE

Answer the following statements true (T) or false (F).

31. T  F  The home health aide is the person who spends the least amount of time with the client.

32. T  F  The client becomes confused; the client was not confused earlier. The home health aide should contact the doctor.

33. T  F  The home where the client lives may be upset before the home health aide arrives; the home health aide should leave if it is too bad.

34. T  F  If the client asks the home health aide to take her to the store shopping, the home health aide should assist her to the car.

35. T  F  The client asks the home health aide to join her for lunch, the aide should politely tell her that this is not allowed by the agency, her role is to assist the client.

36. T  F  All six senses are necessary to assist the home health aide in the role as a health care worker.

37. T  F  It is always better to report something you are not sure of than to not report it.

38. T  F  If it is not written, it did not happen.

39. T  F  Your supervisor is really very busy and should not be bothered with information about the client. The supervisor can read it in the chart.

40. T  F  The chart is a legal record and can be used in a court of law.

## MATCHING

Match each description with the proper sense.

41. _____ Do you hear wheezing? coughing?
42. _____ Is the client's speech slurred?
43. _____ Is the food too salty? too spicy?
44. _____ Do you see frayed electrical cords? wet floors?
45. _____ Is the faucet dripping? Can the client hear the telephone? the doorbell?
46. _____ Does the client have bad breath? Do you smell urine?
47. _____ Does the client feel hot? Does the client's skin feel hot? puffy? rough?
48. _____ Does the food smell bad? Does the bathroom smell unclean?
49. _____ Does the client walk steadily? Do you see any red spots? Does the client's skin look red or sore?
50. _____ Are the sheets dry? Is the water for bathing too hot? too cold?

a. sight
b. hearing
c. touch
d. smell
e. taste

## PRACTICAL EXERCISES

In the following list of items, mark 1 if it needs to be reported to your supervisor or mark 2 if it does not need to be reported your supervisor.

51. _____ The client fell down but was not injured.

52. _____ The telephone does not work.

53. _____ The garbage has not been taken out for a week.

54. _____ The client's daughter dropped off her 2-year-old child for you to watch.

55. _____ The client asks you to work on your day off and asks you not to tell the agency.

56. _____ You notice a large amount of blood in the toilet after the client has used it.

57. _____ The client complains that you are not the regular assistant.

58. _____ The client complains about the brand of dishwashing liquid you purchase.

59. _____ The client requests that you take him or her shopping.

60. _____ The client asks you to wash the dog.

## MULTIPLE CHOICE

Choose the correct answer or answers.

61. When caring for a client in the home, it is expected that you
    a. watch the client's favorite television shows with the client
    b. share your feelings regarding the client's concerns about other family members
    c. will use the client's telephone to take care of your necessary tasks
    d. none of these

62. If the client asks the aide to perform duties that have not been assigned by the case manager, the aide
    a. should do what the client requests
    b. can tell what needs to be done
    c. needs to contact the case manager before proceeding
    d. should refuse to perform these tasks

63. The home health aide should be properly groomed at all times. This includes
    a. clean clothing and shoes          c. polished shoes
    b. trimmed fingernails               d. all of these

64. Important instructions that the home health aide needs to know before taking care of the client include
    a. how and who to report information to
    b. how much the client is paying for the aide's services
    c. what kind of laundry detergent the client uses
    d. how the client was referred to the agency

65. If the client is unhappy with the home health aide, the aide should
    a. leave and go somewhere else
    b. tell the client that she will just have to be satisfied because the aide was assigned to her
    c. try to determine why the client is unhappy
    d. report to the case manager

## DOCUMENTATION EXERCISES

In the following exercises, read the description, then document in the following space, the way you would chart it on the client's chart.

66. You arrive at your client's house and as you walk in you see your client sitting in a chair crying. You ask her what is wrong. She shrugs her shoulders and continues to cry.

---

---

67. You prepare lunch for your client. As he starts to eat, you notice that he is putting a large amount of salt on his food. Your supervisor has instructed you that his food is to be served without any added salt.

---

---

68. You notice your client is feeling warm. You check her temperature. It is 100°F. As you look closely at her, you notice her face is flushed and she feels warm when you touch her.

---

---

# Unit 3 Developing Effective Communication Skills

## SHORT ANSWER/FILL IN THE BLANKS

Complete the following sentences with the correct word or words.

1. Effective _____ may be the most important skill that a care provider can learn.

2. Communication is the successful transmission of a message from one _____ to a second _____.

3. The message is sent by the _____.

4. The message is received by the _____.

5. For communication to successfully take place, the message sent and the message received must be the _____.

6. Praising someone for doing the right thing or for doing something well is called _____ _____.

7. To clearly understand what is meant by the sender of a message, it is important for the receiver to ask for _____.

8. Eye contact, body language, and gestures are examples of _____ _____.

9. Four techniques for improving communication with clients with hearing impairments are:

    a. _____

    b. _____

    c. _____

    d. _____

10. Touching someone is a method of _____ communication.

11. _____ is difficult when there are loud noises or when the receiver is distracted.

12. Offering platitudes, such as "Things will be better tomorrow," is a _____ method of communication.

13. Five tools of effective listening are:

    a. _____

    b. _____

    c. _____

    d. _____

    e. _____

14. Communication in the workplace is essential. The health care worker needs to be able to communicate clearly with coworkers. Three examples of information that the home health aide would need to communicate to coworkers are:

    a. _____

    b. _____

    c. _____

15. The health care worker also must communicate clearly with the client. Three examples of information that the worker needs to communicate clearly to the client are:

    a. _____

    b. _____

    c. _____

16. Four active listening behaviors that are helpful in clear communication include:

    a. _____

    b. _____

    c. _____

    d. _____

## TRUE OR FALSE

Answer the following statements true (T) or false (F).

17. T   F   If the client is talking about a subject that the home health aide finds depressing, it is acceptable for the aide to change the subject.

18. T   F   Passive listening, rushing to answer the speaker before he or she is finished, and interrupting the speaker are all examples of poor listening.

19. T   F   The client is talking about how sad she feels because her arthritis is causing her a great deal of pain. It is appropriate for the home health aide to tell her, "Tomorrow's another day."

20. T   F   Yes/no questions are a good way to show the client that you are interested in the dialogue.

21. T   F   Asking the client to advise you on a personal matter is good because it takes the client's mind off self.

22. T   F   "Why" questions are a way of judging another person.

23. T   F   Paying close attention to the speaker is a good listening skill.

24. T   F   Active listening is a tool that will help the worker become involved in the communication process.

25. T   F   It is acceptable to assume that we know what the speaker is saying.

26. T   F   Paraphrasing what you heard means restating in your own words what the other person has said.

## COMMUNICATION EXERCISES

Write the appropriate response to the following remarks.

27. "You do not have to cook for me today; I want you to take me to the mall instead."

_____

_____

28. " I am not important to anyone anymore; they will all be happy when I die."

_____

_____

29. "I have a terrible feeling that something bad is going to happen."

_____

_____

30. "I know you want to hurry up so that you can go spend time with your friends."

_____

_____

31. "You know that Bertha down the hall, she steals everything I get from my daughter."

_____

_____

32. "I am going to die soon, but nobody will tell me the truth."

_____

_____

33. "I just got a phone call from my son; he has not called me for three months."

_____

_____

34. "My daughter wants to bring her children over for me to watch."

_____

_____

## ABBREVIATION EXERCISES ••••••••••••••••••••••••••••••••••••••••••••••••••••••••••

Next to each phrase, write the appropriate abbreviation.

35. every 3 hours _____

36. twice a day _____

37. nothing by mouth _____

38. intake and output _____

39. hour of sleep _____

40. blood pressure _____

41. every other day _____

42. short of breath _____

43. immediately _____

44. when needed or necessary _____

45. bowel movement _____

46. temperature, pulse, respirations _____

47. by mouth _____

48. without _____

49. complains of _____

50. activities of daily living _____

51. wheelchair _____

52. discontinue _____

53. patient _____

54. every day _____

## MULTIPLE CHOICE ••••••••••••••••••••••••••••••••••••••••••••••••••••••••••••••••••

Choose the correct answer or answers.

55. Many factors could affect receiving messages correctly, these include
    a. hearing loss
    b. distracting noise in the room
    c. depression
    d. all of these

56. Nonverbal communication includes
    a. the words the speaker says
    b. the look on the face of the speaker
    c. the language the speaker speaks
    d. wnone of these

57. If the client has hearing loss, the aide should
    a. speak clearly
    b. use short sentences
    c. write when able to
    d. all of these

58. Examples of close-ended questions include
    a. "Tomorrow's another day."
    b. "I can see you are upset by this."
    c. "Do you want to go outside?"
    d. "Why do you think your son is upset?"

59. Communication requires
    a. speaker
    b. receiver
    c. message
    d. all of these

60. An example of asking for more information is
    a. "I'm interested, tell me more."
    b. "I know that you are upset, but there is nothing I can do."
    c. "Today after we finish with your exercises, I'm going to take you for a walk."
    d. "You look cheerful today."

## LABEL THE DIAGRAM

61. Label the parts of the hearing aid in the diagram, Figure 3-1.

    a. _____

    b. _____

    c. _____

    d. _____

    e. _____

    f. _____

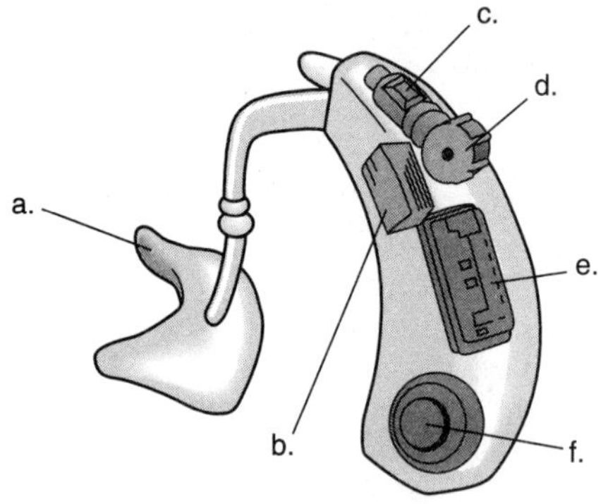

**FIGURE 3-1**

# Unit 4 Safety

## SHORT ANSWER/FILL IN THE BLANKS

Complete the following sentences with the correct word or words.

1. Human factors are directly related to many home _____.

2. Home health aides should be aware of the many causes of accidents in the _____.

3. Some medications make the client unsteady; they may need _____ ambulating.

4. If the client is taking more than one medication, sometimes the medications _____, causing disorientation or unsteady balance.

5. Clients can also become _____ and not remember whether they have taken their medication.

6. According to the National Safety Council, at least one person in _____ suffers some kind of injury as a result of an accident that takes place in someone's home.

7. As the body ages, the bones become brittle and _____ easily.

8. Five ways to make a home a safer environment are:

    a. _____

    b. _____

    c. _____

    d. _____

    e. _____

9. One of the most dangerous rooms in the house is the _____.

10. When transferring a client from or to a wheelchair, the home health aide must remember to _____ _____ _____.

11. Many elderly clients get up at _____ to use the bathroom. It is advisable to keep a _____ on in the bathroom.

12. Elderly persons lose their _____ vision. This means that they can see things _____ _____ only.

13. When a client is wearing a cast, the home health aide should check around the cast frequently for signs of _____ and _____.

14. If the home health aide notices any unsafe conditions in the client's home, the aide should contact the _____ immediately.

15. All homes should be equipped with a _____ _____ in case of fire.

16. If a fire occurs, the home health aide should remember that smoke rises, and if the client cannot be safely moved, the aide should cover the client's face with a _____ _____ and try to move the client to a _____ _____ _____.

17. Smoke rises, and if it is inhaled for a long time, it can cause _____.

18. There are _____ main types of fire extinguishers.

19. If a fire extinguisher is used, it must be held _____ and the nozzle aimed at the _____ edge of the fire.

20. Once a fire extinguisher is used, it must be _____.

21. Five safety tips for the home are:

    a. _____

    b. _____

    c. _____

    d. _____

    e. _____

22. The way in which the body moves and keeps its balance through the use of all its parts is referred to as _____ _____.

23. Medications should be stored out of the reach of _____.

24. To avoid injury to self when caring for a client, the home health aide should always use good _____ _____.

25. The most common injuries for the home health aide involve the muscles, ligaments, and joints of the _____ _____.

26. When you lift, push, or pull, keep your back _____, bend your _____, and use the muscles of your _____ and _____ to do the work.

## TRUE OR FALSE

Answer the following statements true (T) or false (F).

27. T   F   Good body mechanics start with proper posture.

28. T   F   A good standing posture begins with having the feet flat on the floor close together.

29. T   F   Keep your back straight; do not twist or bend.

30. T   F   Hold objects away from your body.

31. T   F   Push, pull, slide, or roll the client whenever possible.

32. T   F   When repositioning the client in bed, turn the client away from you.

33. T   F   When walking with the client, stay on the client's weaker side.

34. T   F   If the client becomes weak while walking with you, let him or her slide to the floor.

## MATCHING

Match the type of accidents with the age group that they are frequently seen in.

35. _____ infants up to 1 year
36. _____ preschool children
37. _____ preteen children
38. _____ teenagers
39. _____ adults
40. _____ old age

a. injuries from motorbikes and autos of carelessness, drunkenness, or drug abuse
b. falls
c. burns from careless use of outside fire and inside fireplace, from overloading electrical circuits, from smoking in bed
d. falls from a table or a bedside
e. scalding from pulling pot handles on stove
f. injuries from bicycle and auto accidents; hit by car when darting into street

## DOCUMENTATION EXERCISES

41. You have taken your client for a walk. She walks using a walker. After she has traveled one block, she becomes very short of breath. After a brief resting period, she is able to walk back to her home. How would you document the walk?

    _____

    _____

42. You are providing care for a bedbound client. The care plan requires that you turn and position him every 2 hours. How would you document this information?

    _____

    _____

43. Your client is unable to transfer from the bed to a wheelchair. You must assist him in this procedure. How would you document this?

    _____

    _____

## Multiple Choice ····················································

Choose the correct answer or answers.

44. Side effects of medication can cause serious problems in clients. _____ should be reported to the case manager immediately.
    a. unusual drowsiness
    b. disorientation and confusion
    c. falling and unsteady ambulation
    d. all of these

45. The most dangerous room in the house is the
    a. kitchen
    b. bedroom
    c. bathroom
    d. garage

46. If the home health aide's clothes start burning, the aide should
    a. run into the shower
    b. stop, drop, and roll
    c. use the fire extinguisher to put out the fire
    d. take off clothing

47. The most common injuries to the home health aide are to the
    a. neck
    b. knees
    c. shoulders
    d. lower back

48. If an injury occurs to a home health aide on the job, the aide should
    a. go to the emergency room immediately
    b. make an appointment to see his or her physician
    c. continue working until the assignment is complete, then report to the supervisor
    d. call and report the injury immediately to the supervisor

## Label the Diagram

49. Label the three elements of the fire triangle in the diagram (Figure 4-1) that are necessary to produce fire.

    a. _____

    b. _____

    c. _____

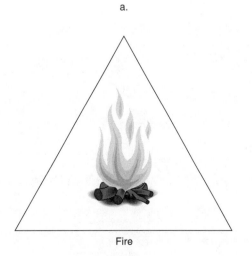

a.

Fire

c.                                                                                                    b.

**FIGURE 4-1**

# Unit 5  Homemaking Service

## SHORT ANSWER/FILL IN THE BLANKS ·············································································

Complete the following sentences with the correct word or words.

1. Managing a household is like operating a daily 24-hour _____.

2. The aide should read directions and ask questions before using unfamiliar _____.

3. Labels should be _____ before using any cleaning product.

4. Wearing _____ will prevent skin irritations caused by soaps or detergents.

5. When handling the client's money, it is always important to get a _____.

6. If a client asks you to perform a task in a different way than you generally perform the task, you should _____ _____ _____ _____.

7. The home health aide should take a few minutes each morning to _____ the day's tasks.

8. Carrying cleaning supplies from _____ to _____ will help make the work go more quickly.

9. Arrange to perform _____ or _____ tasks at one time.

10. Sometimes it is possible to pair household tasks with _____ _____ _____, which helps save time and energy by avoiding many extra steps.

11. Duties that need to be performed each day include:

    a. _____

    b. _____

    c. _____

    d. _____

12. Duties that need to be performed weekly include:

    a. _____

    b. _____

    c. _____

    d. _____

13. Two purposes for changing a bed are:

    a. _____

    b. _____

14. The client, family, and the aide spend more time in the _____ than in any other room.

15. Attractive meals can improve the client's _____.

16. Properly disposing of _____ is extremely important. This will keep the area clean and help prevent disease.

17. If the client has an infectious disease, wash the client's utensils _____ from the other family dishes, then rinse them in _____ _____.

18. Wipe up any spills with a cloth, sponge, or paper towel _____ _____ _____ _____.

19. If blood or other body fluids are spilled on the floor, you must wear _____ and wipe it up with a solution of _____ parts water to _____ part bleach.

20. Cleaning supplies should be stored in a place that is safe from _____ and where confused _____ cannot reach.

21. The natural dampness of the _____ makes it an ideal spot for the growth of mildew and molds.

22. The bathtub needs to be cleaned thoroughly after each _____.

23. Providing nutritious meals requires careful _____.

24. Try to include the _____ and family in the meal planning whenever possible.

25. Always _____ perishable items immediately.

26. Poultry should be _____ before refrigerating.

27. Check food for _____, sour milk, rancid butter, moldy bread, and _____ meats.

## TRUE OR FALSE

Answer the following statements true (T) or false (F).

28. T  F  Never place anything metal in a microwave oven.

29. T  F  Check the label before machine washing garments.

30. T  F  Different colored clothing can be mixed together in the laundry.

31. T  F  It is not necessary to wear gloves when washing clothing of clients infected with the HIV virus.

## DOCUMENTATION EXERCISES

32. You are assigned to care for Mr. Smith. He needs a shower and a meal prepared. When you attempt to assist him to the shower, he tells you he does not feel like taking a shower and he is not hungry. You are aware that the client has a right to refuse care. How would you document his refusal?

_____

_____

33. Your client has an infectious disease. You must wash his dishes separately from other members of the household. How do you document this?

_____

_____

## MULTIPLE CHOICE ·······································································

Choose the correct answer or answers.

34. If the home health aide goes shopping for the client, the aide
    a. should make sure receipts are obtained for all purchases
    b. makes sure to buy the brands that the client requested
    c. gives the appropriate change to the client
    d. all of these

35. Things the home health aide can do to help organize household chores include
    a. making lists of needed supplies and chores to be performed
    b. performing whatever chore looks like it should be done
    c. always making sure the cabinets are closed
    d. wearing rubber gloves to protect hands

36. If the kitchen is kept clean and neat
    a. accidents are less likely to occur          c. germs are less likely to grow
    b. the meals will be easier to prepare          d. all of these

37. When the home health aide handles garbage from the household, the aide
    a. separates the garbage according to local guidelines
    b. double bags the garbage
    c. wears gloves while handling the garbage
    d. all of these

38. The home health aide caring for the toilet needs to remember to
    a. clean the toilet with bleach after each use     c. clean the bathtub with cleanser after each use
    b. clean the mirror after each use                 d. all of these

# Unit 6   Infancy to Adolescence

## SHORT ANSWER/FILL IN THE BLANKS ··································································

Complete the following sentences with the correct word or words.

1. The fertilization of the female egg by the male sperm is called _____.

2. The gestation period is the time from conception to _____.

3. Prenatal care is essential for _____ women.

4. _____ _____ is a surgical technique used to deliver the infant through an incision in the mother's uterus.

5. The process of _____ is an attachment of mother, father, and infant.

6. _____ and _____ are important in the first few months of the infant's life.

7. By age _____ _____, infants can raise their heads and cry when they want to be picked up.

8. Birthweight is usually _____ by 1 year.

9. Babies are born with natural _____; however, after 3 months they need to be protected from illness by vaccines.

10. A DPT vaccine contains _____, _____, and _____.

11. An oral vaccine for _____ is given at 2, 4, and 15 months.

12. A skin test for _____ is given at 1 year.

13. Many states do not allow children to enter school unless they have been properly _____.

14. A common problem with newborns is _____. This means that the child is born before full term.

15. An infant weighing less than _____ pounds is usually considered to be premature.

16. Children born with diseases or malformations need special _____ and _____ care.

17. Jealousy between older children and the new baby is called _____ _____.

18. Children sometimes need help adjusting to the _____ of big sister or big brother.

19. Seven duties the aide must perform for the mother and the newborn are:

    a. _____

    b. _____

    c. _____

    d. _____

    e. _____

    f. _____

    g. _____

20. New mothers need plenty of rest, usually a nap in the _____ and one in the _____.

21. Visitors who have colds or similar infections should not _____ the baby.

22. Ages 1 and 2 are known as the _____ stage.

23. During the toddler stage, the child needs to be watched carefully because the toddler likes _____ _____ _____ _____.

24. Preschool age includes the ages _____ through _____.

25. _____ for achievements is better than punishments for _____.

26. Teenagers have a great need for _____.

27. During _____, the child is strongly influenced by the peer group.

28. During puberty, boys develop _____ on the face and under the arms.

29. Girls develop _____ and _____ and _____ hair.

30. Young girls also begin to _____.

## TRUE OR FALSE

Answer the following statements true (T) or false (F).

31. T  F  Adolescents are hesitant to try new things.

32. T  F  Sex-related problems are especially common in adolescence.

33. T  F  It is estimated that two of five girls now 14 years old will become pregnant before they are 20.

34. T  F  Sexually active teenagers need little guidance in sexual matters.

35. T  F  Substance abuse is a serious problem. It has caused increased crime rate and has destroyed many families.

36. T  F  Religious practices sometimes determine the way birth control is practiced.

37. T  F  Teenagers are aware that alcohol is a dangerous drug.

38. T  F  If parents notice mood swings, red eyes, lethargy, overactivity, sniffling, or other unusual signs, they should seek help for their child.

39. T  F  According to the definition of a "legally responsible person," a home health aide working in the household would not be responsible for reporting abuse.

40. T  F  Abusive parents usually have not been raised by abusive parents themselves.

41. T  F  Life crisis, such as job loss or debt, could cause abuse to a family member.

42. T  F  The home health aide should be aware of the signs of abuse. If the aide becomes aware of them, they need to be reported to the supervisor.

## DOCUMENTATION EXERCISES

43. You are caring for an infant. He has several diarrhea stools. They are liquid and yellow in color. As you change his diaper, you notice his buttocks are slightly reddened. How would you document your observations?

_____

_____

44. You are caring for a client who has recently had a cesarean delivery. She complains of pain in the area of her stitches when she stands.

_____

_____

## MULTIPLE CHOICE

Choose the correct answer or answers.

45. The newborn baby will need the home health aide to
    a. hold and cuddle him or her often
    b. feed him or her whenever he or she cries
    c. assist the mother with bathing the infant
    d. a and c only

46. The home health aide caring for a newborn infant with brothers and sisters needs to
    a. tell the children they cannot touch the baby
    b. encourage the children to help with the care of the infant
    c. allow the children to provide total care for the infant
    d. send the children outside to play while he or she cares for the infant

47. The home health aide assigned to care for a toddler needs to be aware that the toddler
    a. needs to be watched carefully because they are very interested in everything
    b. is learning to talk and walk
    c. needs to be able to explore safely
    d. all of these

48. Adolescence is a difficult time because
    a. many physical and emotional changes are occurring in the youngster
    b. adolescents are just naturally difficult
    c. the adolescent needs special love and understanding
    d. a and c only

49. Teenage pregnancy is a growing problem because of
    a. an increase in sexually active younger teenagers
    b. an increase in sexually transmitted diseases
    c. lack of knowledge of birth control methods
    d. all of these

# Unit 7   Early and Middle Adulthood

## SHORT ANSWER/FILL IN THE BLANKS

Complete the following sentences with the correct word or words.

1. During early adulthood, young adults are concerned with _____ _____.

2. Close personal relationships are _____ during early adulthood.

3. Health problems in early adulthood often accompany _____.

4. A woman should perform a breast self-examination _____, she should have a vaginal examination and a Pap smear performed _____.

5. _____, a rectal examination with a tube, should be performed of both men and women every 3 to 5 years after the age of 50.

6. Middle adult years, ages _____ to _____, are ages when people are expected to be successful and productive.

7. Hormonal changes that occur during menopause may result in _____ _____, changes in _____ patterns, or increased _____.

8. When the grown children leave home, parents sometimes feel a loss. This is called _____ _____ _____.

9. _____ can make anyone old before his or her time.

10. One of the best exercises is _____.

11. As a home health aide, you need to encourage your clients to _____ if they are able to do so.

12. A major crippler of young and middle-age adults is a nervous system disorder called _____ _____.

13. When working with adults who have rheumatoid arthritis, it is better to do exercises _____ in the day.

14. It is very difficult for middle-age adults to accept assistance with _____.

15. Two important needs of persons with disabling conditions are:

    a. _____

    b. _____

16. A major adjustment of most individuals is _____.

17. Retirement from gainful employment may erode one's _____.

## DOCUMENTATION EXERCISES

18. You are caring for a 45-year-old client who is recovering from his first heart attack. He tells you that he does not know what to do: his physician has told him he must take a less stressful job. When you ask him if he is experiencing any pain, he says no but winces every time he moves in bed. How would you document this?

    _____

    _____

19. You are caring for a client who is recovering from a fractured leg. One of your duties is to assist her to the washroom. You do this and she has no difficulty in ambulating with your assistance. Document this.

    _____

    _____

## MULTIPLE CHOICE

Choose the correct answer or answers.

20. Hormonal changes during menopause can result in
    a. graying of the hair
    b. mood swings, hot flashes, increased problems sleeping
    c. the children leaving home
    d. all of these

21. The home health aide needs to be aware of the good effects of exercise, including
    a. problems with stretched muscles
    b. inactivity ages the body
    c. exercise can be called an anti-aging pill
    d. exercise is very time-consuming

22. When caring for a client in this age group (25–65), the home health aide needs to remember that
    a. it is very difficult for these clients to accept assistance from others
    b. these clients are not very grateful at this age
    c. most middle adults will expect you to do everything for them
    d. all of these

23. The disabled client
    a. has the same emotional needs as healthy individuals
    b. generally likes to stay at home
    c. expects more assistance from the home health aide
    d. none of these

24. The main causes of health problems in early adults (25–45) include
    a. problems with arthritis
    b. problems associated with childbirth and accidental injuries
    c. cancer
    d. heart disease

# Unit 8   Older Adulthood

## SHORT ANSWER/FILL IN THE BLANKS

Complete the following sentences with the correct word or words.

1. People become old at different _____.

2. _____ is a process that begins with conception and ends with death.

3. Aged means old or _____.

4. The fastest growing age group in the United States is those over _____.

5. Many older people live alone but still have many _____ and _____.

6. The phenomenon of daughters caring for their aging parents and their own children is called _____ _____.

7. There are some common age-related changes and losses that older people face; however, not all older people experience _____ of the changes.

8. A home health aide working with an older person who is hard of hearing should speak _____ and _____.

9. As people age, many of them have loss of close vision. This can easily be corrected with _____.

10. As America becomes more visual, _____ loss is more difficult to cope with.

11. Urinary incontinence is _____ a part of the normal aging process.

12. Often older people will decrease the amount of _____ they drink each day or not take their "water pill"; both of these acts can have _____ consequences.

13. One thing the home health aide can do to help with urinary incontinence in the elderly is to remind or take the client to the toilet every _____ _____.

14. The home health aide can encourage the client with urinary problems to decrease the amount of _____ consumed because it irritates the bladder.

15. The sense of _____ affects both taste and appetite.

16. The home health aide can help improve _____ by making the food more appealing.

17. Good nutrition can be a challenge for some older people as a result of _____ changes, chronic _____, and obtaining the right _____.

18. Sometimes serving _____ amounts of food more often may make it easier for the client to get the proper nutrition.

19. Breads, cereals, and starches are _____.

20. Tomato products are high in _____ content.

21. Mild exercise done regularly can improve _____, increase _____ mass, and improve _____.

22. The home health aide can go for short walks with the client or assist with exercises only if the _____ allows it.

23. Thinning of bone density caused by loss of bone mass and bone strength is called _____.

24. As we age, sleep is of _____ duration.

25. The elderly take more than _____ of all drugs prescribed in the United States.

26. The home health aide needs to be alert to changes in the client involving _____ or the way _____ is taken.

27. Change is a _____ in life, and if one lives long enough, there is a lot of it.

28. The kind of emotion one feels after a loss or multiple losses can be described as _____.

29. Depression is a persistent _____ that makes it difficult to do day-to-day tasks.

30. Three clues that would lead the home health aide to believe the client is depressed are:

    a. _____

    b. _____

    c. _____

31. The home health aide is one of the persons who sees the elderly client regularly. The aide has the opportunity to identify _____ that could be significant.

32. Many times depression goes _____ in the elderly for a variety of reasons.

33. _____ is a mental deterioration that can involve memory, problem solving, learning, and other mental functions.

34. A home health aide who notices memory loss or confusion must be _____ in raising these concerns with the client.

35. Reminiscence can be a helpful and enjoyable experience for some older people. Five questions that the aide can ask to prompt the client's memory include:

   a. _____

   b. _____

   c. _____

   d. _____

   e. _____

## DOCUMENTATION EXERCISES

36. You enter your client's apartment. Your client, Mrs. Stone, is a 45-year-old woman recovering from a stroke. The first thing you see is her medicine box lying on the floor with all the pills scattered. You ask her what happened. She tells you she does not know. She cannot remember what medicines she has taken. You immediately notify your case manager. How would you document this occurrence?

   _____

   _____

37. You are caring for an 80-year-old client who is very arthritic and a little confused. While you are in the bathroom cleaning the tub, you hear her fall from her chair. After you examine her, you call for assistance because her leg does not look right to you. Document this.

   _____

   _____

## MULTIPLE CHOICE

Choose the correct answer or answers.

38. The home health aide preparing meals for the older person
    a. needs to include well-cooked food
    b. should include a lot of red meat
    c. should offer a variety of foods, including fruits, vegetables, and carbohydrates
    d. none of these

39. The benefits of exercise to the older person include
    a. improved digestion
    b. decreased bone density
    c. increased muscle mass
    d. improved sleep

40. Foods high in sodium include
    a. lemon flavoring
    b. tomatoes
    c. sugar
    d. broccoli

41. Change in the elderly
    a. is a frequent occurrence
    b. involves losses
    c. may result in depression
    d. all of these

42. Age-related mental changes the home health aide can expect to see in elderly clients include
    a. depression
    b. confusion
    c. reminiscence about earlier times
    d. all of these

# Unit 9 Principles of Infection Control

## MATCHING

Match each term with the proper definition.

1. _____ bacteria
2. _____ fungi
3. _____ protozoa
4. _____ pathogens
5. _____ viruses
6. _____ rickettsiae

a. microorganisms that can live only on living cells
b. tiny one-cell microorganisms
c. disease-producing microorganisms
d. microscopic organisms that multiply rapidly
e. a microorganism that lives on lice, ticks, fleas, and mites
f. include yeasts and molds

## SHORT ANSWER/FILL IN THE BLANKS

Complete the following sentences with the correct word or words.

7. The invasion of the body by disease-producing organisms is called _____.

8. Microorganisms are so small, they can only be seen by the use of a _____.

9. Disease-producing microorganisms are called _____.

10. Germs spread rapidly from one part of the body to _____.

11. A home health aide needs to understand how to keep pathogens from _____.

12. The best defense against the spread of _____ is good infection control.

13. Articles that are free of all living things are _____. If the article has any possibility of having germs on it, it is considered to be _____.

14. The process of _____ completely destroys microorganisms.

15. Sterilized supplies must be handled in a special way to prevent them from becoming _____.

16. The process of destroying disease-producing organisms by the use of chemicals is called _____.

17. If two people are using the same stethoscope, the ear pieces must be cleaned with _____ between uses.

18. Three airborne diseases are:

    a. _____

    b. _____

    c. _____

19. Four ways that disease can be transmitted are:

    a. _____

    b. _____

    c. _____

    d. _____

20. Three diseases carried by food are:

    a. _____

    b. _____

    c. _____

21. _____ _____, _____, and _____ are diseases that are transmitted to humans from contaminated drinking water.

22. Two diseases that are transmitted to unborn children by the mother are _____ and _____.

23. When a person steps on a rusty nail, there is a possibility he or she could contract _____.

24. Infectious hepatitis affects the _____.

25. Infectious hepatitis can cause fever, _____, and _____.

26. All home health aides should be _____ against hepatitis.

27. Home health aides taking care of clients with hepatitis should give them good _____ care and _____ care.

28. Tuberculosis (TB) is an _____ disease.

29. The incidence of TB is _____.

30. Individuals most susceptible to TB are persons who live in _____ _____, have _____ _____, are substance _____, are under _____, and lack _____ _____.

31. An aide taking care of a client with TB will need to use _____ _____.

32. Home health aides need to be checked _____ for TB.

33. If the home health aide tests positive for TB, he or she needs to get a _____ _____.

34. Four signs of TB are:

    a. _____

    b. _____

    c. _____

    d. _____

35. It is important for the client with TB to get plenty of _____.

36. Three childhood diseases are:

   a. _____

   b. _____

   c. _____

37. An _____ contracting a childhood disease is affected more seriously than a _____.

38. An aide caring for a sick child needs to practice good infection control techniques to avoid becoming _____.

39. Five common infection control practices include:

   a. _____

   b. _____

   c. _____

   d. _____

   e. _____

40. When people are ill, they _____ fight off other germs.

41. Germs can enter the body in many ways. Four ways are:

   a. _____

   b. _____

   c. _____

   d. _____

42. The most common source of carrying infection are the _____.

43. The most important procedure in controlling the spread of disease is _____ _____.

44. The use of cloth towels can _____ germs.

45. Six times when the hands need to be washed in the client's home are:

   a. _____

   b. _____

   c. _____

d. _____

e. _____

f. _____

## TRUE OR FALSE ··········································································

Answer the following statements true (T) or false (F).

46. T   F   Wash fresh fruits and vegetables before eating or storing them.

47. T   F   After being stored in the cabinet for several weeks, can tops do not need to be cleaned off before opening.

48. T   F   We cannot tell whether people have an infectious disease by looking at them.

49. T   F   It is unnecessary to use standard precautions if you know the client is not contagious.

50. T   F   The client who is feeling isolated or depressed may feel more depressed when the home health aide uses protective barriers such as masks and gowns.

51. T   F   Isolation means the client is kept away from others in the household.

52. T   F   It is unnecessary to wear gloves when emptying a bedpan.

53. T   F   You can wear the moisture resistant gown only once.

54. T   F   All articles used by the client in isolation can be shared with the family.

55. T   F   If blood is spilled on the floor, a preparation of 1 part bleach and 10 parts water must be used to clean it up.

56. T   F   All contaminated materials from the client's room must be discarded by using a special paper or plastic bag and either burning it or placing it in a covered garbage container.

57. T   F   The client's dishes must be washed separately in hot, soapy water; rinsed; and air dried.

## DOCUMENTATION EXERCISES ··········································································

58. You are caring for a client with TB. You are requested to obtain a sputum specimen. You follow the procedure for collecting a sputum specimen. Document the procedure.

_____

_____

59. You are caring for an AIDS client. While you are caring for him, he vomits on the bathroom floor. You clean up the vomitus following correct procedure. Document this occurrence.

_____

_____

## MULTIPLE CHOICE

Choose the correct answer or answers.

60. The home health aide can help prevent the spread of disease by
    a. keeping hands clean
    b. covering nose when sneezing
    c. maintaining good health
    d. all of these

61. Caring for food properly can help prevent the spread of disease. Some things the home health aide can do include
    a. washing fruits and vegetables before eating them
    b. rinsing off the can tops before opening them
    c. cooking meats properly
    d. all of these

62. The home health aide needs to wear gloves when
    a. preparing foods for the client
    b. making the bed of a client
    c. handling body fluids
    d. all of these

63. The home health aide's hands need to be washed
    a. before providing care to a client
    b. before and after putting on gloves
    c. after making the bed
    d. a and b only

## SHORT ANSWER

64. Refer to Figure 9-1. Describe why each item is important in preventing the spread of infection.

    a. _____

    b. _____

    c. _____

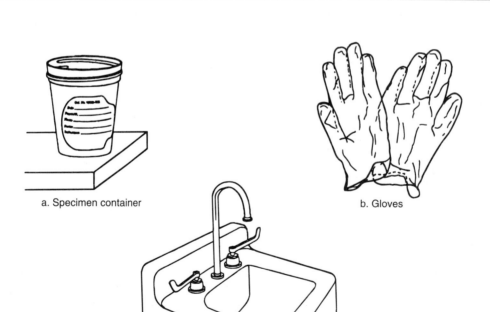

a. Specimen container

b. Gloves

c. Sink

**FIGURE 9-1**

# Unit 10   From Wellness to Illness

## SHORT ANSWER/FILL IN THE BLANKS ·······································································

Complete the following sentences with the correct word or words.

1. _____ is the passing of traits and other individual differences.

2. Environment is the sum total of the circumstances, conditions, and _____ that affect the growth of an organism.

3. Both _____ and _____ contribute to an individual's development.

4. The role of the home health aide is involved in _____ the environment for the client.

5. The human body can adapt to many _____.

6. The smallest structural unit in the body is the _____.

7. _____ occurs when the body is not working properly.

8. External environmental factors that affect the body include _____ and _____.

9. Viruses are external organisms carried through the air in _____ _____.

10. Examples of viruses include _____, _____, and _____.

11. An illness that is sudden and severe is called _____.

12. A chronic illness is one that _____ _____ _____ _____.

13. Illness, an accidental injury, a birth defect, or the normal sensory losses of aging may be the cause of a _____.

14. The Americans with Disabilities Act defines a person with a disability as someone who:

    a. _____

    b. _____

    c. _____

15. It takes longer for recovery in older persons because the growth rate of new cells is _____.

16. A person who normally functions well may have an emotional breakdown when _____ _____ becomes too great.

17. _____ is a normal response to illness.

18. Mentally ill clients need _____ and _____, just as clients with physical problems do.

19. Emotional and physical health are _____ on each other.

20. An emotional illness can cause a _____ illness.

21. Medications can cause _____ or _____.

22. The person who is ill experiences a _____ in physical and emotional energy.

23. Roles in families _____ when a member is ill or becomes disabled.

24. The home health aide must be able to recognize, record, and report significant _____ and _____.

25. A change that can be observed or measured is called a _____.

26. List four signs of a physical change the aide should report to her supervisor.

    a. _____

    b. _____

    c. _____

    d. _____

27. Changes that cannot be observed but are experienced by the client are called _____.

28. Examples of symptoms are:

    a. _____

    b. _____

    c. _____

    d. _____

29. Signs obtained by the use of instruments are called _____ _____.

30. _____ _____ must be measured accurately and regularly.

31. The difference between the heat produced and the heat lost is the body _____.

32. Those clients who cannot hold a thermometer in their mouth must have their temperature taken with a _____ _____.

33. The temperature taken rectally is _____ _____ than the oral temperature.

34. Axillary temperature is _____ the most accurate method for taking a temperature.

35. An axillary temperature is _____ _____ than an oral temperature.

36. The _____ is the artery contracting.

37. Regularity when describing a pulse is described as _____ or _____.

38. The most common site for taking the pulse is the _____ artery.

39. An irregular pulse is one that indicates _____ heartbeats.

40. The strength of the pulse is the force with which the beat is felt. This can be described as bounding, _____, weak, or thready.

41. Pulse rate is described as the number of beats per _____.

42. Normal pulse rates are:

    a. _____ adults

    b. _____ children over 6 years of age

    c. _____ children under the age of 6

    d. _____ infants

43. The amount of force the blood exerts against the walls of the arteries as it flows through them is called _____ _____.

44. The _____ is an instrument used to measure blood pressure.

45. The higher number of the blood pressure reading is called _____; it represents the pressure when the heart is beating.

46. The lower number of the blood pressure reading is called _____; it represents the pressure when the heart is _____ between beats.

47. The _____ number is always recorded first and the _____ number last.

48. If your client has had a stroke, you should take the blood pressure in the arm that _____ _____ _____.

49. If the client has an IV or is receiving _____, you must take the blood pressure in the _____ _____.

50. Two of the greatest potential problems for an unconscious client are _____ _____ and _____.

51. Exercises done to prevent contractures and loss of motion in the joints are called _____ _____ _____.

52. Restoring of physical abilities of the client to the highest level possible is called _____.

53. When the physical ability or skill has been lost, the client must _____.

54. To walk in a partial weight-bearing pattern, the client can use _____ or a _____.

55. The use of a cane requires the client to be _____ weight bearing on both legs.

56. It is important for the home health aide to emphasize the client's _____ rather than _____, when working with a client who is recovering physical ability.

57. The loss of an ability that many of us take for granted is called a _____.

58. _____ are useful in helping a person relearn skills that may have been lost because of the illness or accident.

59. Activities that can help in the rehabilitation process are not limited to arts and crafts but can include:

a. _____

b. _____

c. _____

## MATCHING

Match each term with the proper definition.

60. _____ bradycardia
61. _____ dyspnea
62. _____ apnea
63. _____ respiration
64. _____ rales
65. _____ Cheyne-Stokes
66. _____ rhythm

a. the act of breathing
b. the bubbling sound when fluid gets caught in the air passages
c. slow heartbeat
d. absence of breathing
e. difficult or labored breathing
f. evenness or regularity of the heartbeat
g. respirations that are very rapid, then stop, then start again

## DOCUMENTATION EXERCISES

67. You have checked the vital signs of your client. Temperature is 97.3°F, pulse 86, respirations 18, and blood pressure 126/88. Document these vital signs.

_____

_____

68. You assist your client with walking with a walker. She walks 15 feet, then becomes so tired that she has to rest for 5 minutes. Document this.

_____

_____

69. Your client is spending most of her time in a wheelchair. You try to help her ambulate, but she tells you she prefers to remain in the wheelchair and watch television. You notice a reddened area on her right heel. After you have reported this to your supervisor, how would you document it?

_____

_____

## MULTIPLE CHOICE

Choose the correct answer or answers.

70. Heredity can determine
a. talents and abilities
b. physical wellness
c. height and weight
d. all of these

71. The normal range of rectal temperature in an adult is
a. 96.6°–98.6°F
b. 99.6°–100.0°F
c. 97.6°–99.6°F
d. 94.6°–98.6°F

72. A pulse that skips every fourth beat is called
    a. normal
    b. irregular
    c. faint
    d. bounding

73. The first beat heard in the stethoscope when taking the blood pressure is referred to as the
    a. blood pressure
    b. diastolic
    c. systolic
    d. none of these

74. The client walking with a cane should hold the cane in
    a. the left hand
    b. the right hand
    c. the hand opposite the weak leg
    d. either hand

## LABEL THE DIAGRAM

75. Refer to Figure 10-1. Label the sites where the pulse can be taken.

    a. _____

    b. _____

    c. _____

    d. _____

    e. _____

    f. _____

    g. _____

    h. _____

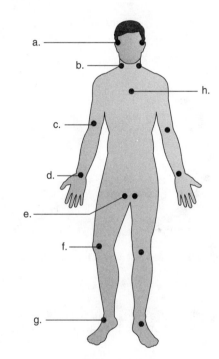

**FIGURE 10-1**

76. Refer to Figure 10-2. Take a reading at the closest line.

    _____

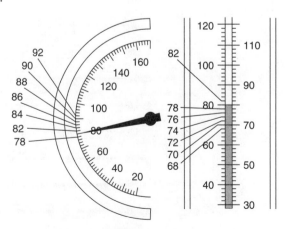

**FIGURE 10-2**

77. Refer to Figure 10-3. Determine the systolic and diastolic readings.

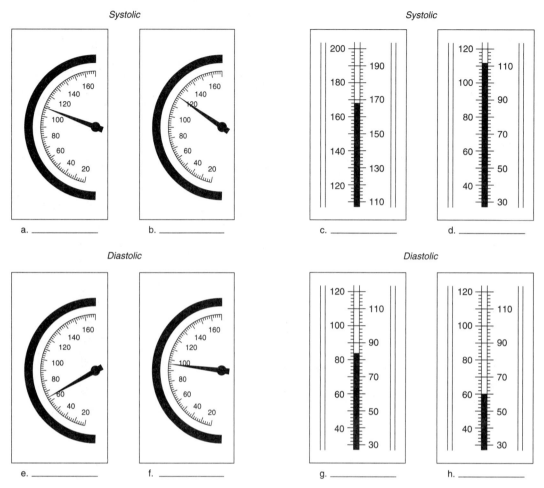

**FIGURE 10-3**

78. Read the following thermometers (Figure 10-4) and write the temperature in the space provided. Be sure to write "F" for Fahrenheit and "C" for Celsius.

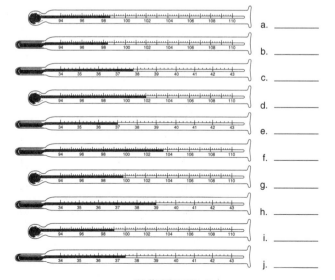

**FIGURE 10-4**

79.  Read the following columns of mercury (Figure 10-5) and write the number in the space provided.

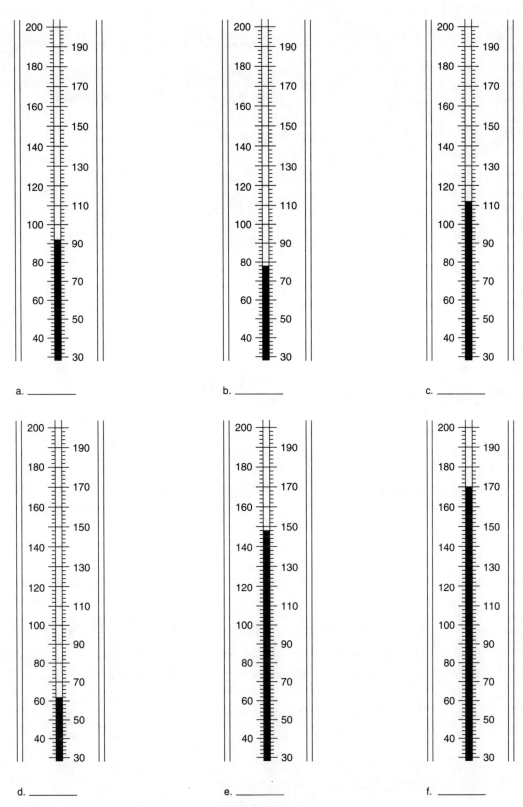

a. _____

b. _____

c. _____

d. _____

e. _____

f. _____

**FIGURE 10-5**

# Unit 11   Mental Health

## SHORT ANSWER/FILL IN THE BLANKS

Complete the following sentences with the correct word or words.

1. The science of human behavior is called _____.

2. An adjustment is the _____ a person makes in behavior to cope with a situation.

3. The well-adjusted individual has a good _____ and can be _____ in new or difficult situations.

4. The body's communication center is the _____.

5. People who are depressed show signs of feeling extremely _____.

6. Depressed persons have difficulty paying _____ and may also be _____.

7. Three negative thoughts caused by depression are:

   a. _____

   b. _____

   c. _____

8. Three physical changes caused by depression are:

   a. _____

   b. _____

   c. _____

9. Depressed people are _____ to control the way they feel.

10. A home health aide needs to listen to the depressed client with _____.

11. The home health aide needs to emphasize doing things _____ the client rather than doing things _____ the client.

12. The home health aide is in a unique position to recognize changes in the client that could indicate signs of _____ thoughts.

13. If the home health aide notices signs that indicate the client is having suicidal thoughts, the aide needs to _____ _____ _____.

## MATCHING

Match each term with the proper definition.

14. _____ internal stimuli
15. _____ external stimuli
16. _____ emotion
17. _____ mental disorder
18. _____ dementia
19. _____ delirium
20. _____ depression
21. _____ psychosis

a. a serious condition in which the thinking process is distorted by hallucinations or delusions
b. a disturbance of consciousness, making it difficult for a person to focus or shift attention
c. emotional blue feelings
d. a strong generalized feeling
e. cause automatic or unconscious reactions within the body
f. loss of intellectual functions
g. difficulty functioning as a result of changes in thoughts, behavior, emotions
h. outside the body stimuli

## DOCUMENTATION EXERCISES

22. You are caring for a 78-year-old lady who recently had cataract surgery. She tells you that she sees a beautiful pink lake with blue fishes swimming all around. How would you document this?

_____

_____

23. You arrive at your client's home. He is sitting in the closet. He tells you to be very quiet because the Germans have landed on the roof. If you make too much noise, they will come down and arrest you. How would you document this?

_____

_____

24. You are caring for a 50-year-old lady whose husband has recently died. You find her staring out the window in her bedroom. She is weeping and tells you there is no point in going on. There is no one who cares for her any longer. Document this.

_____

_____

## MULTIPLE CHOICE

Choose the correct answer or answers.

25. Illness of the client
    a. can cause temporary emotional changes in the client's personality
    b. generally has no effect on the client's personality
    c. can affect the home health aide
    d. none of these

26. The home health aide caring for an emotionally upset client needs to
    a. feel free to have strong outbursts of anger at the client, if it is justified
    b. be able to cope with his or her own emotional needs
    c. be kind and understanding with the emotionally upset client
    d. b and c only

27. Dementia, delirium, depression, and psychotic disorders are examples of
    a. strange ways of thinking
    b. mental disorders
    c. emotions
    d. behavior seen in persons with character disorders

28. Empathy is
    a. sympathy
    b. telling the client that everything will be better tomorrow
    c. telling the client to "snap out of it"
    d. being able to look at the world through the other person's eyes

29. A home health aide caring for a depressed client should
    a. perform all necessary tasks for the client
    b. never leave the client alone
    c. encourage the client to use his or her remaining capabilities
    d. refuse to prepare meals until the client chooses the menu

# Unit 12   Digestion and Nutrition

## SHORT ANSWER/FILL IN THE BLANKS

Complete the following sentences with the correct word or words.

1. The sum of a combination of processes by which the body receives and uses food and nutrients is called
   _____.

2. Those parts of food that cannot be used by the body are expelled as _____ _____.

3. In the body, the fuel is _____; the process of burning this fuel is called _____.

4. Digestion begins in the _____.

5. Food is moved through the esophagus and the stomach by the process of _____.

6. Bile enters the small intestine and breaks up _____ so that they can be absorbed.

7. A condition in which bowel movements are hard and difficult is _____.

8. An elastic, muscular organ that holds the food and secretes and mixes it in gastric juices is called the
   _____.

9. The small intestine consists of the _____, _____, and _____.

10. If the home health aide notices blood in the stool of the client, the aide should _____
    _____ _____ _____.

11. A condition in which feces are watery and frequent is called _____.

12. A backflow of digestive juices into the lower portion of the esophagus, causing irritation to the lining is
    called _____.

13. The professional person who evaluates the client's medical needs and prepares the meal plan is called a
    _____.

14. Indicate in the list below the percentage of each food group recommended in a balanced diet:

_____ fat                                  _____ simple sugars

_____ protein                              _____ carbohydrates

15. Two degenerative diseases are:

   a. _____

   b. _____

16. Early signs of malnutrition are _____ _____ and a constant feeling of _____.

17. As the malnutrition progresses, the symptoms become more severe and include _____ abdomen, a dull film over the _____, hair that is _____ and _____, and bones that become _____.

18. It is generally recommended that a person drink _____ _____ _____ _____ _____ _____ per day.

19. Three reasons to include ample water in the diet are:

   a. _____

   b. _____

   c. _____

20. The home health aide needs to consider the general guidelines for good nutrition when preparing meals for the client, and the aide also needs to consider _____ _____.

21. A service that brings hot meals to homebound persons is called _____ _____ _____.

22. A food allergy is any negative reaction to a food that involves the _____ _____.

23. Three factors to consider when planning a meal for your client are:

   a. _____

   b. _____

   c. _____

24. If your client asks for food that is not allowed on his special diet, what would you tell him?

   _____

   _____

25. Three foods a client on a low-calorie diet should avoid are:

   a. _____

   b. _____

   c. _____

26. A drug called a _____ is given to people with high blood pressure and causes _____ to be flushed from the body.

27. Liquid diets are usually prescribed for people who are recovering from an _____, _____, or _____.

28. The diet prescribed for individuals with difficulties in swallowing is called a _____ diet.

29. Clients with AIDS generally require a diet high in _____ and _____. These clients would benefit from frequent _____ and regular snacks.

30. Experts recommend that the daily intake of _____ be limited to 2,400 to 5,000 mg.

31. Factors affecting high blood pressure are heredity, _____, and excessive drinking of _____.

32. If it is necessary to feed a client, the food will be digested better in a _____ position.

33. Clients who tend to choke easily will choke less if the liquid is _____.

34. Clients who cannot swallow are sometimes fed through a _____.

35. Ask the client which _____ is desired first, when feeding.

36. Three foods excluded from a soft diet are:

    a. _____

    b. _____

    c. _____

37. Four foods included in a diabetic diet are:

    a. _____

    b. _____

    c. _____

    d. _____

38. Three foods excluded from a low-sodium diet are:

    a. _____

    b. _____

    c. _____

39. Three foods you could prepare on a low-fat diet are:

    a. _____

    b. _____

    c. _____

40. Three foods excluded from a diabetic diet are:

   a. _____

   b. _____

   c. _____

41. Three foods you could prepare on a full-liquid diet are:

   a. _____

   b. _____

   c. _____

42. Three foods included on a high-fiber diet are:

   a. _____

   b. _____

   c. _____

43. Three foods to avoid on a low-fiber diet are:

   a. _____

   b. _____

   c. _____

44. Four foods that are high in potassium are:

   a. _____

   b. _____

   c. _____

45. Three functions of vitamin C are:

   a. _____

   b. _____

   c. _____

46. Three sources of vitamin C are:

   a. _____

   b. _____

   c. _____

## MATCHING

Match each term with the proper definition.

47. _____ carbohydrates
48. _____ proteins
49. _____ fats
50. _____ minerals
51. _____ water
52. _____ calorie
53. _____ metabolism
54. _____ vitamins

a. a tasteless, odorless liquid
b. a measure of heat produced by the body when using a specific portion of food
c. organic substances vital to certain metabolic functions and needed to prevent deficiency
d. sum total of processes needed for the breakdown of food and absorption of nutrients
e. sugars or starches that are made up of carbon, hydrogen, and oxygen and deliver quick energy to the body
f. inorganic elements essential in tissue building and in regulation of body fluids
g. compounds composed of amino acids needed for growth and tissue repair
h. oily substances made up of glycerin and fatty acids

## TRUE OR FALSE

Answer the following statements true (T) or false (F).

55. T  F  The average individual should walk 39 minutes a day.

56. T  F  It is important to eat foods from each of the five major food groups each day.

57. T  F  It is acceptable to eat candy and sweet desserts as long as a person is not overweight.

58. T  F  The normal person requires 40 nutrients for good health.

59. T  F  If you take vitamin supplements, you can eat whatever you want.

60. T  F  Whole grain bread and cereals are good sources of fiber.

61. T  F  Milk is a good source of calcium and iron.

62. T  F  Women and adolescent girls need to eat more calcium-rich foods.

63. T  F  Pregnant women generally need an iron supplement.

64. T  F  Most health authorities recommend a diet low in fat and cholesterol.

65. T  F  The risk of heart disease increases in persons who have high cholesterol blood levels, have high blood pressure, and smoke.

66. T  F  Animal fats are not the source of saturated fats in most diets.

67. T  F  To lower cholesterol, you need to eat less animal fat, use oils and fats sparingly, use small amounts salad dressings, and use skim or low-fat dairy products.

68. T  F  Empty calorie foods are foods with no calories.

69. T  F  Calories that are not used by the body are turned into fat for storage.

## DOCUMENTATION EXERCISES ••••••••••••••••••••••••••••••••••••••••••••••••••••••

70. You prepare a meal for your client. He picks at the food and eats only a few bites of the potatoes, a small bite of the meat, and none of the carrots or salad. How would you document his appetite?

_____

_____

71. Your client has been placed on a high-potassium diet. What would you serve him and how would you document it?

_____

_____

## MULTIPLE CHOICE ••••••••••••••••••••••••••••••••••••••••••••••••••••••••••••••••••

Choose the correct answer or answers.

72. Daily food guides recommend
    a. 4–5 servings of meat daily
    b. 2–3 servings of breads daily
    c. 2–3 servings of dairy products daily
    d. 4–5 servings of fats daily

73. The foods highest in vitamin C are
    a. fish, beef, and tuna
    b. citrus fruits, melons, broccoli
    c. cheese, milk, and yogurt
    d. rice, pasta, bread

74. Vitamin $B_{12}$ is essential for
    a. metabolism
    b. healthy red blood cells
    c. treatment of pernicious anemia
    d. all of these

75. Vitamin K is essential for
    a. growth
    b. normal clotting of blood
    c. shiny hair and teeth
    d. none of these

76. Good sources of vitamin D include
    a. spinach
    b. margarine, butter
    c. sunshine, milk
    d. dark green, leafy vegetables

77. Low-sodium diets are usually prescribed for
    a. headaches
    b. diabetes
    c. intestinal problems
    d. heart disease, fluid retention

78. Good sources of calcium are
    a. milk and milk products
    b. red meat and fish
    c. green leafy vegetable
    d. breads and rice

## LABEL THE DIAGRAM

79. Label the sections of the food pyramid with the types of food and number of recommended servings, Figure 12-1.

a. _____     d. _____

b. _____     e. _____

c. _____     f. _____

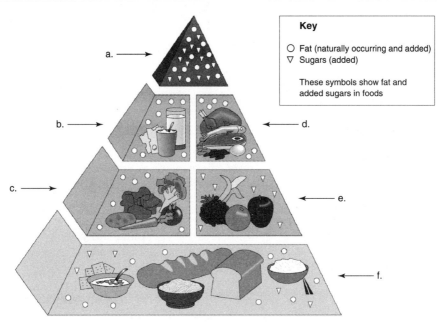

**FIGURE 12-1**

80. Label the parts of the digestive system on the diagram, Figure 12-2.

a. _____

b. _____

c. _____

d. _____

e. _____

f. _____

g. _____

h. _____

i. _____

j. _____

k. _____

l. _____

m. _____

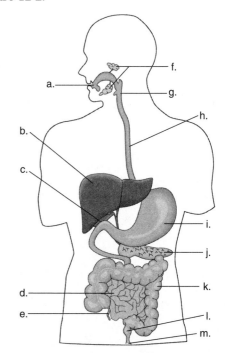

**FIGURE 12-2**

# Unit 13   Elimination

## SHORT ANSWER/FILL IN THE BLANKS

Complete the following sentences with the correct word or words.

1. The urinary system is composed of the kidneys, ureters, _____ and urethra.

2. The primary organs of the urinary system are the _____.

3. The muscular organ for storing urine is called the _____.

4. The normal urine output per day is _____ to _____ mL.

5. Individuals who have lost control of the bladder are referred to as _____.

6. Inflammation of the lining of the bladder is called _____.

7. Incontinence of urine can cause skin _____.

8. Kidney stones can cause _____ urination.

9. A _____ is a tube inserted into the bladder to drain urine.

10. The closed drainage system should _____ be disconnected.

11. A urinary leg bag allows the client greater _____ but must be emptied more often.

12. When the leg bag is not being used, it must be sealed with a clean _____ or _____.

13. The home health aide needs to keep a record of how often and how much a client _____ to learn the client's voiding patterns.

14. Bladder training includes offering the client a specified amount of fluid, and _____ minutes later, the aide should _____ the client.

15. During bladder training, the client needs _____ to remain dry.

16. A common cause of incontinence is _____ in getting to the bathroom.

17. The intervals between toileting may be _____ as control of the bladder is established.

18. An _____ is the technique of introducing fluid into the rectum to remove feces and flatus from the rectum and colon.

19. An _____ contains ingredients that once absorbed by the lining of the colon will stimulate the colon to evacuate stool.

20. Illness, poor eating habits, drug therapy, and lack of exercise can cause _____.

21. _____ is the unusual retention of fecal matter along with infrequent or difficult passage of stony, hard stool.

22. Important elements of a bowel training plan include:

    a. _____

    b. _____

    c. _____

    d. _____

    e. _____

    f. _____

    g. _____

23. A large amount of stool in the lower rectum or colon is called an _____.

24. An impaction must be removed by a _____.

25. To minimize embarrassment to the client in the event of an accident, the client can wear _____.

26. An operation in which the intestine is cut and brought to the outside of the body is called a _____ or an _____.

27. A client with a new colostomy needs the home health aide to be _____ and not show _____.

28. For the home health aide to irrigate a client's _____, the aide needs to have advanced training from the agency.

## DOCUMENTATION EXERCISES

29. You have given your client a fleet enema. His bowel movement was dark brown and very hard. He passed some flatus and stated he felt much better. Document this occurrence.

    _____

    _____

30. Your client is incontinent of urine frequently. She uses five to six diapers a day. How would you document this?

    _____

    _____

31. You have been asked to collect a urine specimen from your client. You have collected it. Document it.

    _____

    _____

## MULTIPLE CHOICE ··················································

Choose the correct answer or answers.

32. Actions the home health aide can take to help the client who is constipated include
    a. encouraging fluid intake
    b. increasing fiber in diet
    c. encouraging exercise
    d. encouraging the use of laxatives

33. The purpose of caring properly for an ostomy bag is to
    a. keep the client clean
    b. prevent skin breakdown
    c. regulate daily routine for removing wastes
    d. all of these

34. The home health aide monitoring intake for a client needs to measure
    a. coffee
    b. cream
    c. sugar
    d. toast

35. Measures the home health aide can perform to prevent skin breakdown in the incontinent client include
    a. keeping the perineal area clean and dry
    b. applying moisture barrier ointment
    c. inspecting the affected area frequently
    d. changing the diaper at least once a day

36. When the membrane lining the bladder becomes inflamed, _____ occurs.
    a. incontinence
    b. cystitis
    c. kidney stones
    d. none of these

## LABEL THE DIAGRAM ··················································

37. Label the parts of the urinary system on the diagram, Figure 13-1.

    a. _____

    b. _____

    c. _____

    d. _____

    e. _____

    f. _____

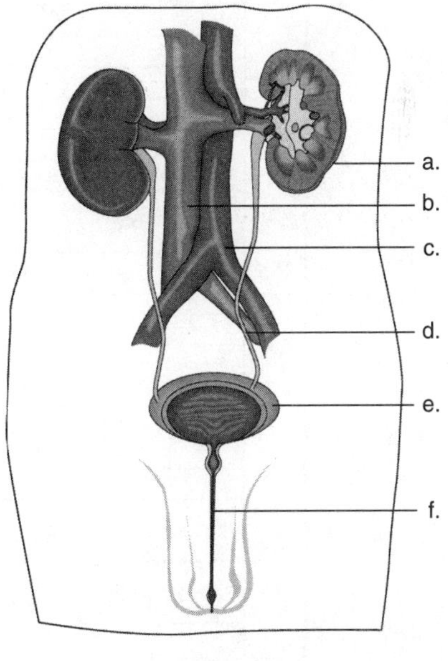

**FIGURE 13-1**

38. Record the following day of oral intake on the form provided in Figure 13-2. The following cups, bowls, and glasses are used in the facility:

| | |
|---|---|
| juice glass | 150 mL |
| bowl | 250 mL |
| coffee cup | 200 mL |
| carton of milk | 240 mL |
| custard, ice cream, and gelatin | 125 mL |

Intake Section of Intake and Output Form

| Time | Oral | | Tube Feeding | Intravenous | Other |
|---|---|---|---|---|---|
| | Kind | Amount | | | |
| | | | | | |
| | | | | | |
| | | | | | |
| | | | | | |
| | | | | | |
| | | | | | |
| | | | | | |
| | | | | | |
| 8-Hour Total | | | | | |
| | | | | | |
| | | | | | |
| | | | | | |
| | | | | | |
| | | | | | |
| | | | | | |
| | | | | | |
| | | | | | |
| 8-Hour Total | | | | | |
| | | | | | |
| | | | | | |
| | | | | | |
| | | | | | |
| | | | | | |
| | | | | | |
| | | | | | |
| | | | | | |
| 8-Hour Total | | | | | |
| 24-Hour Total | | | | | |

**FIGURE 13-2**

39. Indicate with a yes or no which areas could be contaminated, Figure 13-3.

a. _____

b. _____

c. _____

d. _____

e. _____

f. _____

g. _____

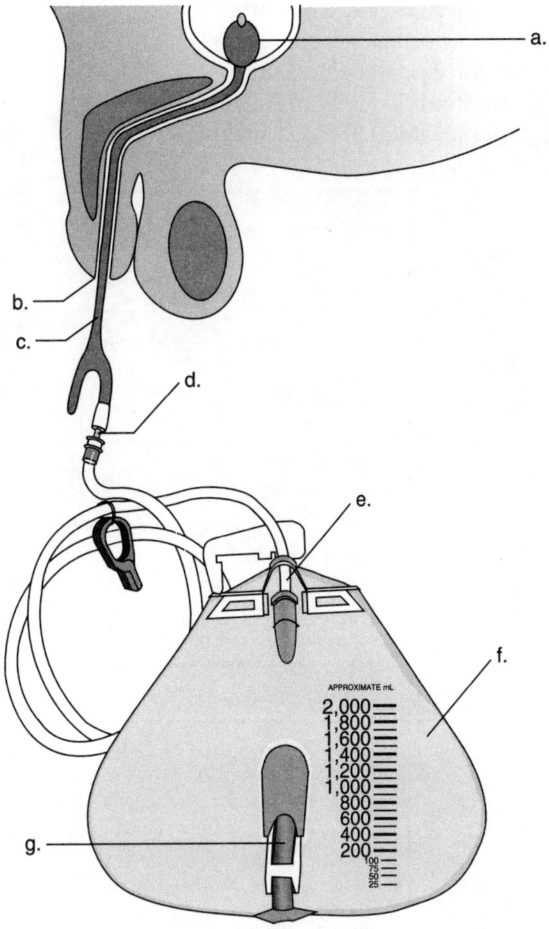

**FIGURE 13-3**

40. Use the following measurements to fill out the urinary output portion of the I&O form, Figure 13-4.

0630 patient voided 450 mL urine
0900 patient voided 200 mL urine
1330 patient voided 345 mL urine
1615 patient voided 280 mL urine
2220 patient voided 370 mL urine

Output Section of Intake and Output Form

| OUTPUT | | | | |
|---|---|---|---|---|
| Time | Urine | Emesis | BM | Other/Kind |
| | | | | |
| | | | | |
| | | | | |
| | | | | |
| | | | | |
| | | | | |
| | | | | |
| | | | | |
| 8-Hour Total | | | | |
| | | | | |
| | | | | |
| | | | | |
| | | | | |
| | | | | |
| | | | | |
| | | | | |
| 8-Hour Total | | | | |
| | | | | |
| | | | | |
| | | | | |
| | | | | |
| | | | | |
| | | | | |
| 8-Hour Total | | | | |
| 24-Hour Total | | | | |

**FIGURE 13-4**

# Unit 14   Integumentary System

## SHORT ANSWER/FILL IN THE BLANKS ·······························

Complete the following sentences with the correct word or words.

1. The integumentary system is made up of the skin, _____, and _____.

2. Skin is made up of two layers: one is called the _____ and the other layer is called the _____.

3. Three functions of the skin are:

   a. _____

   b. _____

   c. _____

4. The natural openings in the skin are called _____.

5. Secretions from the glands help keep _____ from entering the pores.

6. The pus that forms on a skin wound is made up of _____ _____ _____.

7. Three ways that hair protects the body are:

   a. _____

   b. _____

   c. _____

8. Pressure areas on the body are sometimes called _____.

9. A person who gets little exercise and spends most of the time lying in the same place can expect to experience _____ _____.

10. Skin breakdown is most likely to occur over _____ _____.

11. Five areas of the body that are likely to experience skin breakdown are:

   a. _____

   b. _____

   c. _____

   d. _____

   e. _____

12. Describe the four stage of pressure sores.

    a. _____

    b. _____

    c. _____

    d. _____

13. The home health aide needs to reposition the bedbound client every _____ _____ to prevent skin breakdown.

14. Four components of good skin care that the home health aide must perform are:

    a. _____

    b. _____

    c. _____

    d. _____

15. Two conditions that may occur when the environmental conditions are extreme and the person's skin is unable to regulate body temperature are _____ and _____.

16. Six signs of hyperthermia are:

    a. _____

    b. _____

    c. _____

    d. _____

    e. _____

    f. _____

17. If you are caring for a client and he shows any of the above signs and his temperature is elevated, what steps would you take?

    a. _____

    b. _____

    c. _____

    d. _____

    e. _____

18. _____ is a condition marked by an abnormally low internal body temperature.

19. Four signs of hypothermia are:

   a. _____

   b. _____

   c. _____

   d. _____

20. Good hygiene is an important to maintain _____ integrity, prevent _____, and to re-fresh and _____ the client.

21. The home health aide should check the client's skin for any signs of _____ when giving a bath.

22. The purposes of giving the client a bed bath include cleaning the client, _____ _____, and observing the body for signs of _____ _____.

23. A back rub is given to increase the blood _____ to the back and to provide _____ and _____ to the client.

24. The area from the genitals to the anus is called _____.

25. Good oral hygiene is important to keep the client's _____ and _____ healthy.

## TRUE OR FALSE

Answer the following statements true (T) or false (F).

26. T   F   The skin is the largest organ of the body.

27. T   F   When the air evaporates the perspiration on the body surface, the skin temperature rises.

28. T   F   The home health aide needs to inform the supervisor when the client's skin breakdown has reached a stage three.

29. T   F   If the client is left lying in an urine soaked bed, the skin break down will occur rapidly.

30. T   F   If the client is lying in a bed with an air mattress, it is not necessary to turn the client every 2 hours.

31. T   F   Older people are less likely to die from heat-related causes than younger people.

32. T   F   An older person may be reluctant to run air conditioners because of the cost.

33. T   F   If your client is experiencing hypothermia, you should wrap him or her in a warm blanket.

34. T   F   It is a good idea to use electric heating pads set on high and placed on the client's abdomen.

35. T   F   It is a good idea to offer the client the bedpan before giving a bath.

36. T   F   Keeping the perineum clean is important to prevent infection.

## MATCHING

Match each term with the proper definition.

37. _____ air mattress
38. _____ egg crate
39. _____ sheepskin
40. _____ gel foam
41. _____ heel pads
42. _____ water mattress

a. a barrier between the client's skin and the sheets
b. a mattress filled with air
c. a special cushion filled with a solution or gel
d. a mattress filled with water
e. a foam rubber mattress
f. special protectors for the heel

## DOCUMENTATION EXERCISES

43. Your client has a wound on his lower left leg. You are required to perform a dressing change. You notice the wound is approximately 1 inch in diameter and is a very dark red. You apply antibiotic ointment and a sterile $4 \times 4$, and tape to secure. Document this.

_____

_____

44. Caring for your client includes giving a bed bath, making the bed, and transferring the client into a wheelchair. How would you document his care?

_____

_____

45. When you arrive to care for Mr. Moon, you find him sitting outside in the sun. The weather is very hot. He tells you that he feels terrible. He is dizzy, nauseated, and feels very weak. His skin is very dry, and he has chest pain. After you call for help, what do you document?

_____

_____

## MULTIPLE CHOICE

Choose the correct answer or answers.

46. Areas of the body especially prone to skin breakdown include
    a. bony prominences
    b. areas covered with hair
    c. urine-soaked areas
    d. a and c only

47. Special devices that can help prevent skin breakdown include
    a. cane
    b. walker
    c. wheelchair
    d. sheepskin, elbow and heel pads

48. The home health aide performing dressing changes needs to document the
    a. size of the wound
    b. color of the drainage
    c. color of the bandage used
    d. a and b only

49. The purpose of giving the client a bed bath is to
    a. provide exercise for the aide
    b. put the client at ease
    c. clean and refresh the client
    d. give the client an opportunity to talk

50. The bedpan should be offered
    a. before bathing
    b. after eating
    c. before ambulating the client
    d. all of these

## LABEL THE DIAGRAM

51. Refer to Figure 14-1 and draw a circle around ten areas at risk for the development of pressure ulcers.

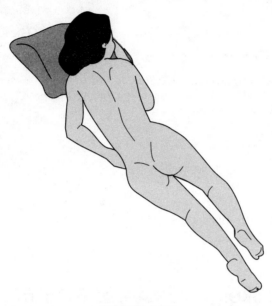

**FIGURE 14-1**

52. Indicate with a yes or no whether the diagram shows the correct taping, Figure 14-2.

    a. _____

    b. _____

    c. _____

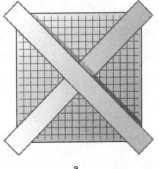
a.

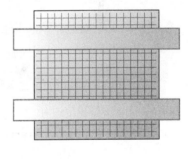
b.

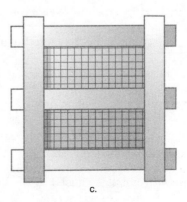
c.

**FIGURE 14-2**

53. Label the parts of the integumentary system, Figure 14-3.

a. _____

b. _____

c. _____

d. _____

e. _____

f. _____

g. _____

h. _____

i. _____

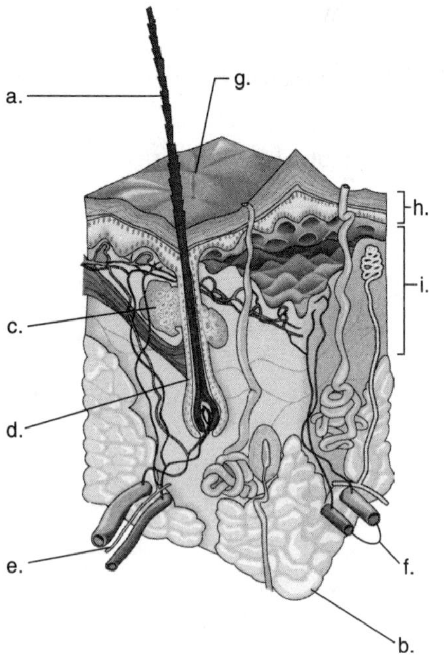

**FIGURE 14-3**

# Unit 15    Musculoskeletal System: Arthritis, Body Mechanics, and Restorative Care

## SHORT ANSWER/FILL IN THE BLANKS

Complete the following sentences with the correct word or words.

1. The musculoskeletal system is made up of _____ and _____.

2. The musculoskeletal system protects the internal _____ _____ and makes _____ possible.

3. A protective covering for the brain is called the _____.

4. Tough elastic fibers that hold the bones together are called _____.

5. The _____ allow the bones to be moved in certain ways.

6. The elbow and knees have hinge joints, which move only in _____ direction.

7. Joints at the shoulder and pelvis are _____ and _____ joints—they allow circular movement.

8. A break in a bone is called a _____.

9. Muscles whose movement is caused by the brain are called _____ muscles.

10. A condition that affects the bone joints and produces painful, swollen joints is called _____.

11. The most painful time of day for clients with arthritis is the _____.

12. A type of arthritis that affects mainly men is called _____.

13. Arthritis is managed with _____ therapy, an _____ program, surgery, and _____.

14. Clients with arthritis may have lack of appetite because of _____.

15. If the client is experiencing pain in the joints, it is a good idea to remind the client to take pain medicine ½ hour before performing _____.

16. Decreased activity may cause the arthritic client to _____ weight.

17. Impaired _____ may cause lack of energy for preparing foods and shopping by the client with arthritis.

18. Aspirin is the drug of choice for arthritis, but sometimes it causes problems with the person's _____.

19. The client who uses many over-the-counter medications to treat arthritic pain should be encouraged to contact his or her _____ regarding medications.

20. Many times the client with arthritis can be helped by _____.

21. Assistive devices are used to maintain _____, simplify _____, and minimize _____ to the joints.

22. Correct positioning of the body can make the client _____ and assist the body to _____ more efficiently.

23. Casts are used to immobilize _____ or joints after trauma.

24. In caring for clients with casts, you examine the cast for signs of _____ that may cause skin irritation.

25. Four symptoms of rheumatoid arthritis are:

    a. _____

    b. _____

    c. _____

    d. _____

26. Four symptoms of osteoarthritis are:

    a. _____

    b. _____

    c. _____

    d. _____

# TRUE OR FALSE

Answer the following statements true (T) or false (F).

27.  T   F   There are more than 200 bones in the body.

28.  T   F   Involuntary muscles are controlled by the brain.

29.  T   F   The interior of the bone produces new blood cells for the circulatory system.

30.  T   F   The heart is an example of a voluntary muscle.

31.  T   F   Involuntary muscles form the walls of organs, these muscles work automatically.

32.  T   F   Arthritis is seen more often in the elderly.

33.  T   F   Arthritis affects 50% of the people over the age of 65, and men are affected twice as often as women.

34.  T   F   Rheumatoid arthritis affects all ages.

35.  T   F   Arthritis is a chronic degenerative disease.

36.  T   F   Exercises that the client can perform without assistance are referred to as passive exercises.

37.  T   F   The goal of an exercise program includes maintaining joint movement or increasing joint movement.

38.  T   F   If the client with arthritis has an exercise program, it is important for the program to be followed by the client even if it is painful.

39.  T   F   It is important for the aide to be able to position the body correctly.

40.  T   F   If the client with a cast develops a crack in the cast, the aide should tape it with adhesive tape.

41.  T   F   If the client complains of itching under the cast, the aide should blow hot air from a hair dryer into the cast.

42.  T   F   Heat applications can increase circulation to a body part.

# DOCUMENTATION EXERCISES

43.  You are assigned to Mrs. Howe, who has rheumatoid arthritis. You are instructed to give her a partial bed bath, allowing her to perform as much as she is able to. When you give her the bath, she is only able to bathe her face and hands. Document her care.

_____

_____

44.  You are assigned to ambulate Mrs. Geever, perform range of motion exercises to the lower extremities, and assist her to the bedside commode. Mrs. Geever complains of severe pain in her shoulder when you are assisting her to her bedside commode. She urinates a small amount and you return her to bed. Document your care and observations.

_____

_____

# MULTIPLE CHOICE ································································

Choose the correct answer or answers.

45. Surgery for arthritis can be performed on the following joints
    a. knee, hip, jaw
    b. spine, shoulder, finger
    c. hip, spine, wrist
    d. all of these

46. You assist the client to a sitting position. You need to check to see that
    a. the client has good body alignment
    b. the client can see the TV
    c. the clothes are clean and neat
    d. the client is relaxed

47. When you are making an occupied bed, you
    a. take all the sheets off before putting clean sheets on the bed
    b. ask the client to get out of the bed
    c. work on only one side of the bed at a time
    d. hurry through changing the bed so that you can get on with other tasks

48. Positioning clients in the Fowler's position
    a. helps assist them to breathe easier
    b. makes it easier for them to get out of bed
    c. allows you to change the bed easier
    d. none of these

49. During the procedure of transferring the client to a wheelchair, you
    a. press your knee against the client's stronger knee
    b. set the chair at a 90° angle to the bed
    c. press your knee against the client's weakest knee
    d. keep your feet together and flex your knees and hips

# LABEL THE DIAGRAM ································································

50. Label the parts of the muscular system on the diagram, Figure 15-1.

    a. _____

    b. _____

    c. _____

    d. _____

    e. _____

    f. _____

    g. _____

    h. _____

    i. _____

    j. _____

    k. _____

    l. _____

    m. _____

    n. _____

    o. _____

    p. _____

    q. _____

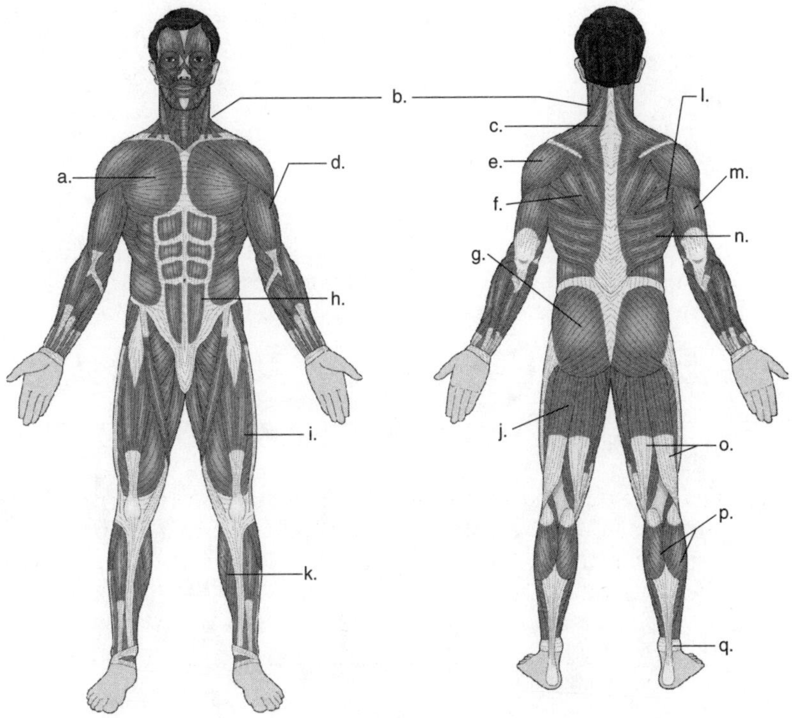

**FIGURE 15-1**

51. Review Figure 15-2.  Choose the word for the range of motion being performed:
    a. rotated
    b. adducted
    c. flexed
    d. abducted

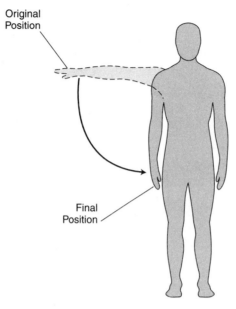

**FIGURE 15-2**

52. Review Figure 15-3.  Choose the word for the range of motion being performed:
    a. abducted
    b. adducted
    c. flexed
    d. rotated

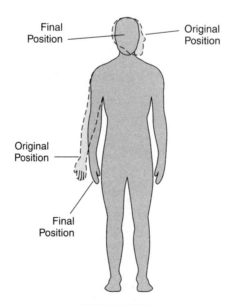

**FIGURE 15-3**

53. Review Figure 15-4.  Choose the word for the range of motion being performed:
    a. rotated                           c. flexed
    b. adducted                          d. abducted

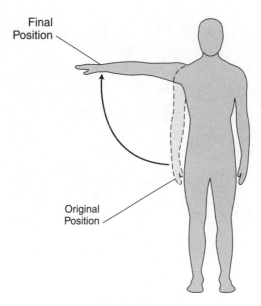

Final Position

Original Position

**FIGURE 15-4**

54. Review Figure 15-5.  Choose the word for the range of motion being performed:
    a. rotated                           c. abducted
    b. flexed                            d. adducted

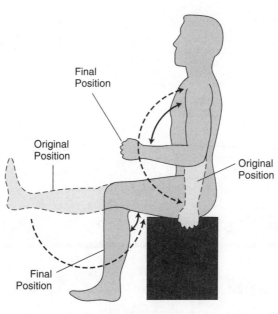

Final Position

Original Position

Original Position

Final Position

**FIGURE 15-5**

55. Label the parts of the skeletal system on the diagram, Figure 15-6.

a. _____

b. _____

c. _____

d. _____

e. _____

f. _____

g. _____

h. _____

i. _____

j. _____

k. _____

l. _____

m. _____

n. _____

o. _____

p. _____

q. _____

r. _____

s. _____

t. _____

u. _____

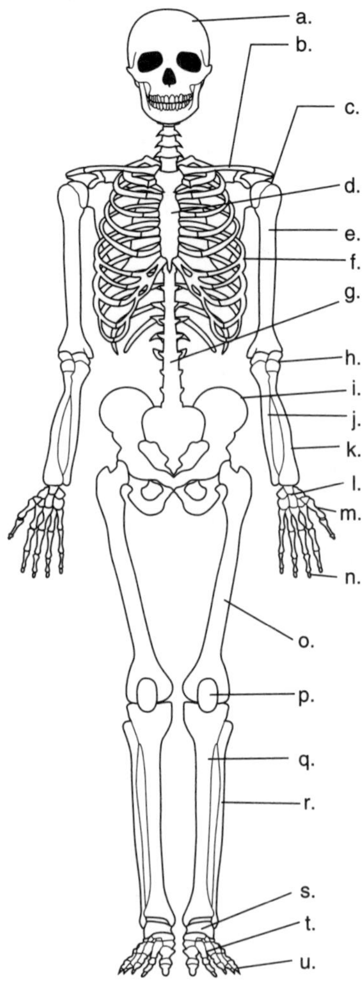

FIGURE 15-6

# Unit 16   Nervous System

## SHORT ANSWER/FILL IN THE BLANKS

Complete the following sentences with the correct word or words.

1. The nervous system is made up of the _____, _____ _____, and
   _____.

2. The five senses are _____, _____, _____, _____, and _____.

3. The spinal cord is protected by the _____ _____.

4. The master switch of the nervous system is the _____.

5. A progressive degenerative disease characterized by shaking, fixated facial expression, shuffling gait, stiffness of limbs, and stooped posture is called _____ _____.

6. The time it takes to respond to a stimulus is called _____ time.

7. Three disorders of the nervous system are:

   a. _____

   b. _____

   c. _____

8. A disease affecting the central nervous system that begins with episodes that only last a short time is _____ _____.

9. Seizures can be caused by many causes. Three causes are:

   a. _____

   b. _____

   c. _____

10. Muscular dystrophy is a progressive disease characterized by muscle _____, lack of _____, inability to lift _____ _____ _____ _____ _____, and progressive _____.

# TRUE OR FALSE

Answer the following statements true (T) or false (F).

11. T   F   The nervous system can be referred as the communication network of the body.

12. T   F   If the spinal cord is cut, the body could still feel the parts below the cut.

13. T   F   The brain alerts other parts of the body and gives them instructions on how to respond to stimuli.

14. T   F   The nerve endings can be compared with electrical outlets.

15. T   F   ALS is another name for Lou Gehrig's disease.

16. T   F   There is no cure for muscular dystrophy.

17. T   F   Loss of hearing or vision affects only older people.

## MATCHING

Match each term with the proper definition.

18. _____ paraplegia
19. _____ quadriplegia
20. _____ hemiplegia
21. _____ brain
22. _____ nerves
23. _____ nervous system
24. _____ CVA
25. _____ seizure
26. _____ otosclerosis
27. _____ cataracts

a. paralysis of one side of the body
b. stroke
c. communication center of the body
d. a cloudy area in the lens of the eye
e. the control center of the nervous system
f. paralysis of both arms and legs
g. involuntary muscular contractions with loss of consciousness
h. paralysis of the lower part of the body
i. affects the bones of the middle ear
j. part of the nervous system that receives stimuli

## DOCUMENTATION EXERCISES

28. You are caring for a client who has had a stroke. While you are bathing her, she starts to have a seizure. She convulses for 2 minutes. You quickly turn her to her side and gently hold her on the bed until she stops convulsing. After the seizure has stopped, she goes to sleep. You notice she has wet the bed. You call and report this to your supervisor. How would you document this?

_____

_____

29. When you arrive at your client's home, you find him sitting on the couch waiting for you. He wants to go to the grocery store and shop. You have been given specific instructions to bathe him and prepare a meal. You know the physical therapist is due to work with him in about an hour. You know that he dislikes his therapy treatments. How would you handle this situation and how would you document it?

_____

_____

## MULTIPLE CHOICE

Choose the correct answer or answers.

30. Medications for the client with Parkinson's disease may cause serious side effects. The home health aide should watch for
   a. frequent urination
   b. constipation
   c. involuntary movements, dizziness, nausea
   d. none of these

31. During a seizure, the home health aide should
   a. roll the client to the side
   b. not limit the movements of the client
   c. loosen clothing
   d. all of these

32. The nervous system is composed of
   a. the lungs and heart
   b. the long bones and small bones of the wrist
   c. the brain, spinal cord, and nerves
   d. none of the these

33. If the spinal cord is damaged, the client will be
   a. hemaplegic
   b. paraplegic
   c. quadriplegic
   d. none of these

## LABEL THE DIAGRAM ································································································

34. Label the parts of the nervous system in the diagram, Figure 16-1.

a. _____

b. _____

c. _____

d. _____

e. _____

f. _____

g. _____

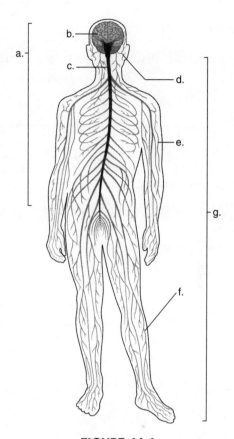

**FIGURE 16-1**

# Unit 17   Circulatory System

## SHORT ANSWER/FILL IN THE BLANKS ····················································

Complete the following sentences with the correct word or words.

1. The organ that supplies power to the body system is the _____.

2. The _____ atrium receives blood from the tissues.

3. The _____ ventricle pumps the blood to the lungs, where it picks up _____.

4. The _____ ventricle pumps the blood out to all parts of the body.

5. The blood carried away from the heart to the body cells in blood vessels called _____.

6. Tiny blood vessels between the arteries and the veins are called _____.

7. The veins carry the blood back to the _____.

8. The pulse measured at the wrist is an expansion of the _____ _____.

9. Arterial blood is _____ _____ in color; this is due to its oxygen content.

10. Venous blood is darker in _____ because of its low oxygen content.

11. Three changes that occur in the circulatory system as a person ages are:

    a. _____

    b. _____

    c. _____

12. Many people become very _____ when they are told they have heart disease.

13. Lack of blood supply to the heart muscle is called _____.

14. A person having an episode of angina pectoris will become _____ and _____. The blood pressure will _____. They will have a mild pain that radiates from the chest to the _____ arm. The client will become flushed and _____. Immediate treatment for angina is _____.

15. A common emergency medication for angina is _____. It can be taken under the _____ or in the form of a patch placed on the skin. The home health aide may have to assist the client in placing the new patch on the skin. The skin should be cleansed thoroughly before the client _____ _____.

16. If the client does not get relief from pain with the nitroglycerin within 15 minutes, the aide should _____ _____ _____.

17. A myocardial infarction is more commonly known as a _____ _____.

18. A myocardial infarction is a condition when the blood vessel of the _____ _____ is blocked, which causes _____ to the heart muscle.

19. Smaller vessels sometimes take over the work of the blocked _____. This is referred to as collateral circulation.

20. Emergency care is needed for the client. The person may go into _____ _____.

21. During a cardiac catheterization, a tube is passed into the heart to detect _____.

22. _____ are drugs that thin the blood and slow the clotting time. The home health aide needs to observe the client who is taking this medication for signs of bleeding. Two signs the aide needs to watch for are _____ and _____; if they occur, the aide needs to _____ _____ _____ _____.

23. Three things the home health aide taking care of the client with congestive heart failure needs to remember are:

    a. _____

    b. _____

    c. _____

24. A condition in which the arteries become hard and lose their elasticity is _____.

25. The home health aide must _____ apply heat to a client's cold feet if the client has arterioscle-rosis. Instead the client should be offered more _____.

26. Pressure sores are caused by poor _____ to a particular area of the body.

27. The client who is unable to move about must be protected from _____. The aide may need to use a bed _____ or a footboard.

28. It is important to _____ the client in bed every _____ _____ if the client is unable to move about in bed.

29. Once a brain cell is destroyed, it _____ be brought back to life.

30. Interruption of blood flow to the brain can be caused by an _____, an _____, or a _____.

31. _____ is important because it helps train the remaining cells of the brain to take over the func-tion of some of the dead brain cells.

32. Four conditions that are associated with increased risk of stroke are:

    a. _____

    b. _____

    c. _____

    d. _____

33. The majority of strokes occur in persons over the age of _____.

34. The home health aide needs to recognize signs of impending stroke. Four signs are:

    a. _____

    b. _____

    c. _____

    d. _____

35. If the aide notices any of these signs of impending stroke, the aide needs to _____ _____ _____.

36. If the client starts showing a deterioration of mental judgment, confusions, memory loss, poor judgment, and personality changes, the client may be developing multiple _____ _____.

37. Cerebral hemorrhage means there is bleeding into the _____.

38. Stroke can affect people in many ways depending on what part of the brain cells are affected. Five deficits resulting from stroke are:

    a. _____

    b. _____

    c. _____

    d. _____

    e. _____

39. The person having a stroke usually _____ consciousness and becomes _____ of bladder and _____. The client's breathing will become _____, and he or she may have a severe _____, slurred _____, and blurred _____.

40. The client usually has weakness on _____ of the body after a stroke.

41. The home health aide can expect the client to have difficulty in speaking, _____, swallowing, and _____.

42. The aide needs to be patient and allow the client to be as _____ as possible after a stroke.

43. The aide may need to assist the client in performing active or passive _____ _____ _____.

44. The client with _____ aphasia can not express himself or herself correctly.

45. In communicating with an aphasic client, the home health aide should ask questions that require a _____ _____.

46. If the client complains of aching in the legs, has edema of the legs, and the legs are discolored, the client could be experiencing venous insufficiency. The aide needs to report these complaints to the _____ _____.

47. Thrombophlebitis is a serious condition. If the client has tenderness, warmth or _____ in the calf of the leg, the aide should report it to the case manager _____.

48. A life-threatening condition that is a complication of thrombophlebitis is _____ _____.

49. Arterial insufficiency is a condition that is caused by narrowing of the _____ that supply the lower extremities. When the client walks or exercises, the leg muscles may become _____.

50. Signs of compete obstruction include severe _____, pallor, absence of _____ in lower leg, numbness, and _____ of the limb.

51. Death of the body tissue caused by lack of adequate blood supply is called _____.

52. A hereditary disease characterized by spontaneous bleeding due to a lack of a clotting factor in the blood is called _____.

# TRUE OR FALSE ............................................................................................

Answer the following statements true (T) or false (F).

53. T   F   Men have a greater risk of having a heat attack than women before menopause.

54. T   F   As people grow older, they have less chance of having a heart attack.

55. T   F   Persons whose parents had heart problems will have a greater chance of having heart disease them-selves.

56. T   F   Persons with high cholesterol levels in their blood have less chance of heart disease.

57. T   F   As stress increase in a person's life, so does the risk of heart attack.

58. T   F   Persons who are overweight, smoke, or have diabetes are at risk for heart disease.

59. T   F   Increasing exercise is a good way to increase the risk of heart attack.

60. T   F   The home health aide is very important in the care of the client who has heart disease.

61. T   F   The effects of nitroglycerin generally occur within 2 to 3 hours.

62. T   F   A CABG is an operation commonly performed on the heart.

63. T   F   A cardiac arrest is a very serious occurrence.

64. T   F   Congestive heart failure is a heart condition that can cause swelling of the legs or feet or fluid in the lungs.

65. T   F   Pressure sores usually are not difficult to heal.

66. T   F   Brain cells die when they do not receive oxygen for more than 4 minutes.

67. T   F   Ambulating the client with a gait belt requires the aide to stand on the client's strongest side.

68. T   F   Retraining the bladder requires the bedpan to be offered at the time and at the same intervals.

69. T   F   A client with receptive aphasia can understand what someone says.

70. T   F   Inflammation of the lining of the vein is called phlebitis.

71. T   F   Sickle cell anemia is seen in African Americans and is a disease where the red blood cells become shaped like a sickle.

72. T   F   A condition in which there are too many red blood cells produced by the body is called leukemia.

## MATCHING

Match each term with the proper definition.

73. _____ CVA
74. _____ aneurysm
75. _____ embolism
76. _____ thrombus
77. _____ atherosclerosis
78. _____ TIA
79. _____ cerebral infarction
80. _____ arteriogram
81. _____ aphasia

a. a blood clot that forms inside an artery
b. stroke
c. x-rays of blood flow in arteries
d. a brief period of weakness, loss of speech or feeling
e. a moving blood clot
f. hardening of the artery
g. ballooning out of the wall of an artery
h. impaired ability to speak
i. a condition in which a portion of the brain dies

## DOCUMENTATION EXERCISES

82. Your client has recently been discharged from the hospital. She had a heart attack. Her physician ordered her to start mild exercising. You have been told to walk her around the apartment twice during your time with her. When you approach her with the walker, she becomes very upset and states, "The doctor is trying to kill me. I know if I walk around this room, I will have another heart attack and die." What do you do to calm her down? How will you get her to ambulate? Document this information.

_____

_____

83. Mrs. K. is your second client of the day. She has a diagnosis of angina. You are running about 20 minutes later than usual. When you arrive, she is agitated. She grasps her chest and tells you she has been having chest pain all morning. What will you do first? After a short time, she calms down and allows you to assist with her bath. Do you contact your supervisor? Document this information.

_____

_____

## MULTIPLE CHOICE

Choose the correct answer or answers.

84. Signs of side effects of anticoagulants include
    a. bleeding from the gums
    b. bruises on the extremities
    c. all of these
    d. none of these

85. To prevent the client who is unable to swallow well from choking, the home health aid should
    a. check the mouth after eating to see if food remains caught in the paralyzed side
    b. check to see if the client has been incontinent
    c. offer the bedpan
    d. speak clearly to the client

86. The home health aide caring for the client with a blood clot in her leg should encourage the client to
    a. ambulate with a walker
    b. walk with the cane on the weaker side
    c. use crutches
    d. remain in bed

87. The home health aide caring for a client with elastic stockings should
    a. ask the client to sit in a chair while the aide applies the stockings
    b. apply the stockings while the client is lying down
    c. reapply the stockings each day
    d. none of these

## LABEL THE DIAGRAM ·················································

88. Label the parts of the cardiovascular system, Figure 17-1.

a. _____

b. _____

c. _____

d. _____

e. _____

f. _____

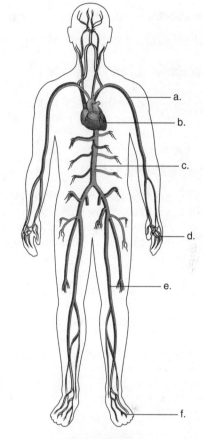

**FIGURE 17-1**

89. Label the parts of the circulatory system, Figure 17-2.

a. _____

b. _____

c. _____

d. _____

e. _____

f. _____

g. _____

h. _____

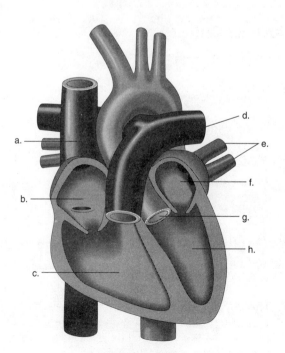

**FIGURE 17-2**

# Unit 18 Respiratory System

## SHORT ANSWER/FILL IN THE BLANKS

Complete the following sentences with the correct word or words.

1. The respiratory system keeps the body supplied with _____.

2. Oxygen is carried by the blood to the cells of the body. At the same time, _____ _____ is picked up from the cells by the blood and taken to the lungs where it is removed from the body.

3. Pneumonia is an infection of the _____. It is the _____ cause of death in the United States.

4. The _____ are particularly susceptible to pneumonia. The home health aide needs to be alert to the symptoms to alert the nurse.

5. Chronic bronchitis can result from asthma, bronchitis, _____ _____, and _____ _____.

6. Bronchitis is inflammation of the _____.

7. Four symptoms of bronchitis are:

   a. _____

   b. _____

   c. _____

   d. _____

8. Medications are given to the client with bronchitis to dilate the _____ and facilitate _____ _____.

9. A condition caused by an allergic reaction is _____.

10. Asthma is associated with _____of large and small airways.

11. Client experiencing an asthma attack feel anxious and _____.

12. The home health aide needs to help the client with respiratory distress to relax and remain _____.

13. A lung condition in which the air sacs within the lung lose their elasticity is called _____.

14. The typical emphysema client is a _____, 50 to 60 years of age.

15. The client receiving oxygen therapy needs to have _____ mouth care.

## DOCUMENTATION EXERCISES ·······················································

16. You are instructed to care for Mr. L. When you arrive to bathe him, you find him sitting in a chair. He is chain smoking and has an oxygen cannula in his nose. You see a plastic tube that runs from his nose into the next room. In the next room, you locate his oxygen concentrator. You remind him that it is not safe to smoke around oxygen. He states it is safe because the oxygen is in the next room. What would do? How would you document this information?

_____

_____

17. You are asked to obtain a sputum specimen from your client. Document this procedure.

_____

_____

## MULTIPLE CHOICE ·······················································

Choose the correct answer or answers.

18. Clients with chronic respiratory difficulties will need
    a. a soft, comfortable chair
    b. a box of Kleenex
    c. frequent rest periods
    d. none of these

19. The role of the home health aide in breathing treatments includes
    a. preparing the medication
    b. instructing the client in the proper technique
    c. administering the breathing treatment
    d. observing the client for difficulties with the treatment

20. Pneumonia is dangerous to the elderly because
    a. they have many chronic diseases
    b. the elderly are more vulnerable
    c. both a and b
    d. none of these

21. Structures of the respiratory include the
    a. heart and veins
    b. lungs, nose, and trachea
    c. kidneys, heart, and sinuses
    d. all of these

22. Assisting the client with deep breathing exercises includes asking the client to
    a. take deep breaths through the nose
    b. hold the breath for 5 to 7 seconds
    c. take a deep breath and cough
    d. all of these

23. The home health aide's role in oxygen therapy includes
    a. instructing people not to smoke around oxygen
    b. giving the client frequent mouth care
    c. applying lubricant to lips
    d. all of these

## LABEL THE DIAGRAM ••••••••••••••••••••••••••••••••••••••••••••••••••••••••••••••

24. Label the parts of the respiratory system, Figure 18-1.

a. _____

b. _____

c. _____

d. _____

e. _____

f. _____

g. _____

h. _____

i. _____

j. _____

k. _____

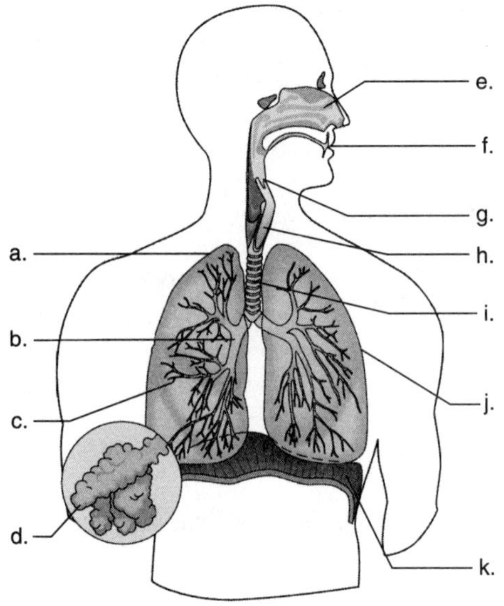

**FIGURE 18-1**

# Unit 19   Reproductive System

## SHORT ANSWER/FILL IN THE BLANKS ••••••••••••••••••••••••••••••••••••••••••••••

Complete the following sentences with the correct word or words.

1. The male reproductive organs are the _____ and the _____.

2. The female reproductive organs are the _____ and _____.

3. The mouth of the uterus is called the _____.

4. Menstruation is the sloughing off of the uterine _____. This occurs every _____ days if the egg is not fertilized.

5. The _____ that produce male and female characteristics are also thought to help maintain function in other systems of the body.

6. The pain females experience with menstruation is called _____.

7. Vaginitis can be caused by bacteria, protozoa, or _____.

8. _____ usually has a white discharge with intense itching and burning.

9. Treatment for reproductive illnesses should by started only after the client has seen a _____.

10. Pelvic inflammatory disease can result in _____.

11. A pregnant female with gonorrhea risks passing the illness to the _____.

12. Gonorrhea cause _____ from the penis.

13. The earliest symptom of _____ is an ulcer.

14. Late effects of syphilis include disorders of the brain, _____, and _____.

15. _____ is a common STD and it tends to recur.

16. The first attack of herpes may be accompanied by _____, fever, and pain in the _____, _____, and _____.

17. Persons with herpes can relieve the symptoms with _____ _____ and _____ _____.

18. Persons with the symptoms of STD should _____ from sex. Their _____ should be checked for infection.

## TRUE OR FALSE

Answer the following statements true (T) or false (F).

19. T   F   Sexually transmitted diseases are spread by causal contact.

20. T   F   STDs have become more prevalent in recent years.

21. T   F   Pelvic inflammatory disease is generally a result of an STD.

22. T   F   There is no cure for herpes.

23. T   F   Sexually active persons should practice safe sex.

## DOCUMENTATION EXERCISES

24. You are assigned to care for Mr. Jon, who has recently had a catheter placed into his bladder. While you are bathing him, you notice urine on the bed sheet. What do you need to do? How do you document this finding?

_____

_____

25. Your client, Mr. Tote, has a diagnosis of genital herpes. You are required to give Mr. Tote a bed bath; he is unable to assist you. You know that you need to wear gloves and follow good universal precautions. How do you document this care?

_____

_____

## MULTIPLE CHOICE

Choose the correct answer or answers.

26. Pelvic inflammatory disease can be caused by
    a. pneumonia
    b. gonorrhea
    c. chlamydia
    d. both b and c

27. Small blisters on the penis and around the vagina are symptoms of
    a. herpes
    b. gonorrhea
    c. AIDS
    d. none of these

28. There is no cure for
    a. AIDS
    b. gonorrhea
    c. syphilis
    d. pneumonia

29. Pain that sometimes accompanies menstrual flow is called
    a. vaginitis
    b. gonorrhea
    c. dysmenorrhea
    d. nausea

## LABEL THE DIAGRAM

30. Label the parts of the male reproductive system on the diagram, Figure 19-1.

    a. _____

    b. _____

    c. _____

    d. _____

    e. _____

    f. _____

    g. _____

    h. _____

    i. _____

    j. _____

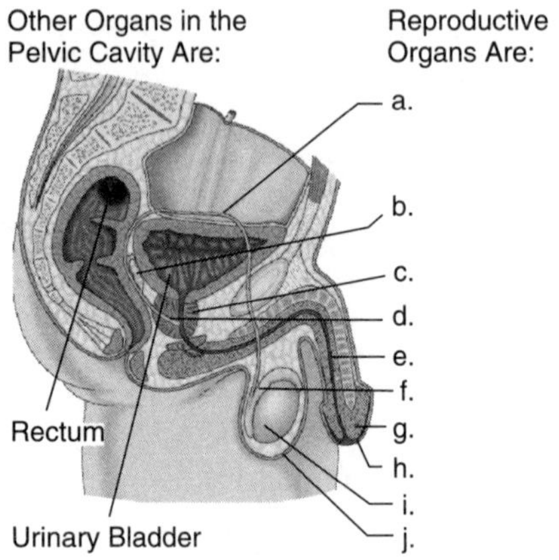

Other Organs in the Pelvic Cavity Are:

Reproductive Organs Are:

a.
b.
c.
d.
e.
f.
g.
h.
i.
j.

Rectum

Urinary Bladder

**FIGURE 19-1**

31. Label the parts of the female reproductive system on the diagram, Figure 19-2.

    a. _____

    b. _____

    c. _____

    d. _____

    e. _____

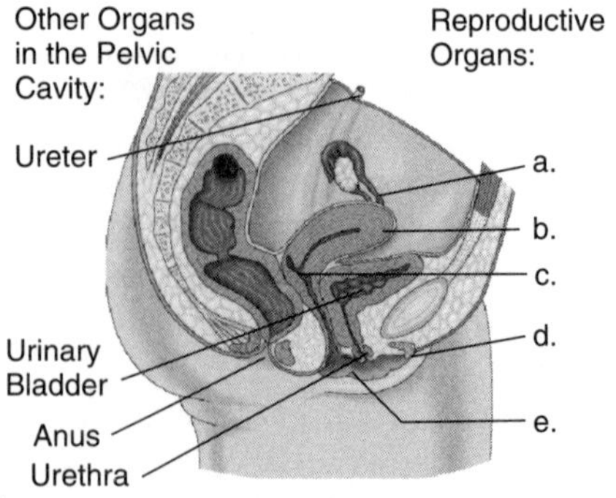

Other Organs in the Pelvic Cavity:

Reproductive Organs:

Ureter

a.
b.
c.
d.
e.

Urinary Bladder

Anus

Urethra

**FIGURE 19-2**

32. Label the parts of the female reproductive system on the diagram, Figure 19-3.

a. _____     e. _____

b. _____     f. _____

c. _____     g. _____

d. _____

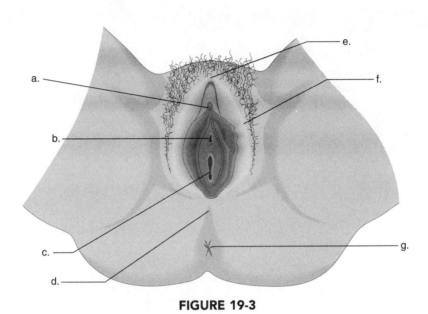

**FIGURE 19-3**

# Unit 20   Endocrine System and Diabetes

## SHORT ANSWER/FILL IN THE BLANKS

Complete the following sentences with the correct word or words.

1. Substances that are secreted by the endocrine glands are called _____.

2. These secretions are carried by the blood or lymph system to all parts of the body to _____ and _____ body functions.

3. The _____ regulates the metabolic rate of the body.

4. Persons with hyperthyroidism have a _____ heartbeat and tend to be _____.

5. Persons with an underactive thyroid tend to be sluggish and _____ _____ easily.

6. The function of insulin is to enable the body to use _____.

7. Diabetes develops when _____ is not produced by the body.

8. The build up of sugar in the blood causes difficulty in _____.

9. Five symptoms of diabetes are:

   a. _____

   b. _____

   c. _____

   d. _____

   e. _____

10. Testing for diabetes can be done on either _____ or _____.

11. The home health aide needs to be alert to signs of _____ and _____ and also needs to be able to follow the emergency plan for the client if either of the two occurs.

12. Signs of hypoglycemia include _____, _____, _____ _____, _____, and _____ _____ _____ _____.

13. Signs of hyperglycemia include _____ _____, _____ _____, _____, _____ _____, and _____ and _____.

14. When the blood sugar reaches above 300, a serious condition called _____ occurs. The aide needs to call for emergency help.

15. Loss of vision is a frequent complication of _____.

16. _____ is the keystone to the management of diabetes.

17. The diet needs to contain _____% to _____% carbohydrates, _____% to _____% protein, and _____% to _____% fats.

18. Exercise can improve the client's _____, assist in maintaining _____, increase the client's sense of _____, and improve control of _____ in the body.

19. The home health aide plays an important role with the diabetic client by _____ him or her to comply with requirements for exercise, especially if the client is discouraged.

20. Insulin cannot be taken orally because the stomach juices will _____ it.

21. A home health aide is _____ permitted to inject insulin.

22. The home health aide can help the client by bringing the bottle of _____ to the client.

23. A new device for injecting insulin over time is called the insulin _____.

24. Diabetes type II can be treated in three ways. The three ways are:

   a. _____

   b. _____

   c. _____

25. As home health aide, it is important to encourage the client to take the medicine as it is _____.

26. Neuropathy is defined as a destructive disorder of the _____.

27. Neuropathy is the loss of sensation in the _____.

28. It is important for the home health aide to check the client's _____ every time the aide provides care to make sure there are no wounds or injuries.

29. Trimming the toenails of a diabetic client must be performed by a _____.

30. The diabetic client's feet must be cleansed with a mild _____, _____, and lotion applied.

31. Clients with diabetes are very susceptible to _____.

32. The risk of infection in the diabetic client is increased because the high _____ in the blood helps bacteria to grow.

33. The bed linens need to be _____, _____, and _____.

34. The client needs to be _____ and _____ every 2 hours if confined to bed.

35. Hot and reddened areas of the skin are the first sign of _____.

# TRUE OR FALSE

Answer the following statements true (T) or false (F).

36. T   F   Hormones are powerful substances.

37. T   F   Adrenalin causes the heart to slow down.

38. T   F   Diabetes is the third leading cause of death in the United States.

39. T   F   More than 11 million people in the United States have diabetes and almost half of them do not know it.

40. T   F   Insulin-dependent diabetes usually occurs after the age of 25.

41. T   F   Chinese Americans have a high rate of non–insulin-dependent diabetes.

42. T   F   Sometimes pregnant women develop diabetes.

43. T   F   Exercise, alcohol, or decreased kidney functions can make hypoglycemia worse.

44. T   F   The normal blood sugar levels are between 60 and 250.

45. T   F   Improperly treated diabetes can lead to complications.

46. T   F   Walking barefoot in the house is okay for diabetic clients, as long as they are careful.

47. T   F   When the aide bathes the feet of the diabetic client, the water must be warm and not hot.

48. T   F   It is a good idea for the diabetic client to wear a medic alert tag.

49. T   F   A diabetic client who develops acidosis, or insulin shock, needs to be informed to call his physician for an appointment.

## DOCUMENT EXERCISES

50. Mrs. Macy, your client, has diabetes and recently had to have an amputation of her lower left leg. When you arrive, you find her in the kitchen. She is eating sweet rolls. You greet her and ask her if the sweet roll is dietetic. She tells you that she is allowed to eat sweet rolls as long as she does not put sugar on them. What would you do? How would you make her understand that foods that have sugar in them do not always look like they do?

_____

_____

51. Mrs. Tam is an insulin-dependent diabetic. She has been diabetic for a short time. You are caring for her because she recently fractured her leg and needs help bathing. She informs you that she has been vomiting all night and is concerned that you will have to clean up the mess. She says, "I took my insulin just like I was supposed to." What do you say to her? Do you need to report this information to your case manager? Why? Document this.

_____

_____

## MULTIPLE CHOICE

Choose the correct answer or answers.

52. The gland called *master gland* is the
    a. thyroid
    b. adrenal
    c. pituitary
    d. thymus

53. The function of insulin is to help the body
    a. fight infection
    b. use sugar
    c. grow in height
    d. none of these

54. The type of diabetes that occurs during pregnancy in some women is called
    a. gestational
    b. insulin-dependent
    c. non–insulin-dependent
    d. all of these

55. Signs and symptoms that may indicate diabetes include
    a. frequent urination
    b. excessive thirst
    c. sores that do not heal
    d. all of these

56. Foods that the diabetic client should avoid or eat in small amounts include
    a. green leafy vegetables
    b. citrus fruit juices
    c. cakes and candies
    d. both b and c

## LABEL THE DIAGRAM ••••••••••••••••••••••••••••••••••••••••••••••••••••••••••

57. Label the endocrine glands in the diagram, Figure 20-1.

a. _____

b. _____

c. _____

d. _____

e. _____

f. _____

g. _____

h. _____

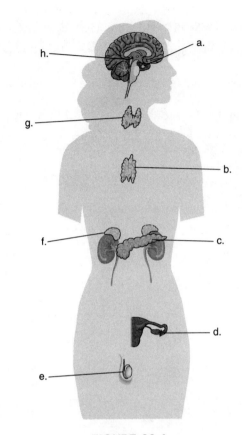

**FIGURE 20-1**

58. Label the parts of the endocrine system in the diagram, Figure 20-2.

a. _____

b. _____

c. _____

d. _____

e. _____

f. _____

g. _____

h. _____

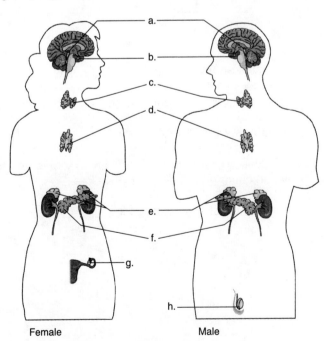

Female                                    Male

**FIGURE 20-2**

# Unit 21   Caring for the Client Who Is Terminally Ill

## SHORT ANSWER/FILL IN THE BLANKS

Complete the following sentences with the correct word or words.

1. Most people in our society are uncomfortable with _____.

2. Families are now allowing their loved ones to die at _____.

3. The goal of _____ is to keep the client comfortable and as pain free as possible.

4. Native Americans used to leave their loved ones alone to _____.

5. The Patient Self-Determination Act is a law passed to allow clients to make a decision about the use of _____ _____.

6. Advanced directives can be done by a living _____ or by a durable power of _____.

7. The home health aide needs to respect the family's _____ in dealing with the death of a loved one.

8. Signs of approaching death include:

    a. _____

    b. _____

    c. _____

    d. _____

    e. _____

    f. _____

9. The client should be treated with _____ and _____ at all times.

10. It important for the home health aide to remain _____ when death occurs.

11. A death that is sudden is more _____ than one following a long illness.

12. Religious practices differ from person to person, the aide needs to become _____ with the family and client practices.

13. Death is usually the cause of a _____ within the family.

## MATCHING

Match each term with the proper definition.

14. _____ denial
15. _____ anger
16. _____ bargaining
17. _____ depression
18. _____ acceptance

a. calmly facing what is to be
b. "Dear God, I'll be good. Please not yet."
c. "This can't be happening to me."
d. feeling that this death is unfair; bitterness
e. brooding, withdrawal, "I cannot go on living."

## TRUE OR FALSE

Answer the following statements true (T) or false (F).

19. T   F   Some of the medical advances prolong life but do not improve life.

20. T   F   The home health aide should offer advice to the client or family of the dying client.

21. T   F   The unconscious client can still hear what is being said.

22. T   F   Good communication skills are important when working with the dying client and family.

23. T   F   The most difficult time for the family after the death of a loved one is the first 2 or 3 months.

## DOCUMENTATION EXERCISES

24. You have been caring for Mr. Howe for a week. He had a stroke and has been unconscious since. You are aware that the physician thinks that he is not going to recover. His daughter greets you as you walk in to care for him. She tells you that he moves in his sleep and that she knows now that he will recover. What will you tell her? You know that many times unconscious persons move but that particular movement is a neurological reaction. You want to reassure her but you know that he is not expected to improve.

_____

_____

25. When you arrive to care for Mr. Howe, you notice that he has noisy, labored respirations and his pulse is very weak and irregular. You feel that death is approaching. What do you document? Will you take his vital signs? What will you tell his relatives?

_____

_____

## MULTIPLE CHOICE

Choose the correct answer or answers.

26. The last sense to be lost in a dying person is
    a. sight
    b. hearing
    c. touch
    d. smell

27. The hospice program accepts clients that generally have
    a. less than 1 year to live
    b. less than 3 months to live
    c. cancer
    d. 6 months to live

28. The five stages of dying were first described by
    a. Einstein
    b. Bill Clinton
    c. Dr. Kübler-Ross
    d. The Patient Self-Determination Act

# Unit 22  Caring for the Client with Alzheimer's Disease

## Short Answer/Fill in the Blanks

Complete the following sentences with the correct word or words.

1. Alzheimer's disease is a _____ _____ disease that attacks the brain.

2. This disease is characterized by loss of _____ and diminished _____ _____.

3. Five symptoms of Alzheimer's disease are:

   a. _____

   b. _____

   c. _____

   d. _____

   e. _____

4. Ten warning signs of Alzheimer's disease are:

   a. _____

   b. _____

   c. _____

   d. _____

   e. _____

   f. _____

   g. _____

   h. _____

   i. _____

   j. _____

5. If the client becomes upset about something, try to _____ him or her with something else.

6. The home health aide caring for an Alzheimer's client must have a great deal of _____, _____ and _____ of the disease process.

7. The family caring for a relative with Alzheimer's disease needs to have times of _____ away from the client.

8. Four things the home health aide can do to assist the client in communication are:

   a. _____

   b. _____

c. _____

d. _____

9. The home health aide needs to take the Alzheimer's client to the bathroom _____ .

10. The home health aide should be aware of possible side effects of any _____ the client is taking.

11. If the client exhibits disruptive behavior, the home health aide should try to determine the _____ of the behavior.

12. Validation therapy is used to increase _____ and _____ feelings.

13. These clients have little short-term memory, but many _____ memories remain.

14. Exploring memories of the past with the client is called _____ .

15. Ten tips for communicating with the client with dementia are:

a. _____

b. _____

c. _____

d. _____

e. _____

f. _____

g. _____

h. _____

i. _____

j. _____

## TRUE OR FALSE

Answer the following statements true (T) or false (F).

16. T   F   Alzheimer's disease is the third leading cause of death in the adult population.

17. T   F   The identified risk factors for Alzheimer's disease are family history and age.

18. T   F   The time from onset to death can range from 3 to 20 years in Alzheimer's disease.

19. T   F   There is a specific test for Alzheimer's disease.

20. T   F   People with Alzheimer's are usually happy and cheerful.

21. T   F   If you forget the food cooking on the stove, you probably have Alzheimer's disease.

22. T   F   Consistency is extremely important when caring for clients with Alzheimer's disease.

23. T   F   Clients with Alzheimer's cannot control their behavior.

24. T   F   The client with Alzheimer's disease sleeps for many hours without interruption.

25. T   F   Playing soft, soothing music helps calm the agitated client.

26. T   F   Wandering is the most common agitated behavior among people with Alzheimer's disease.

27. T   F   If the client starts to wander, the aide should try to stop him or her.

## DOCUMENTATION EXERCISES

28. When you arrive at the home of Mrs. Lee, she runs out the door past you. You know that her diagnosis is Alzheimer's disease. You also know that she likes to wander around the neighborhood. It is very cold outside, and she is dressed only in a nightgown. What will you do first? Will you take her for a walk? Document your interventions.

_____

_____

29. After you have dressed Mrs. Lee and taken her for a walk, you try to feed her. She spits the food at you. You know that this is typical behavior for Mrs. Lee. What can you do to distract her?

_____

_____

## MULTIPLE CHOICE

Choose the correct answer or answers.

30. The only identified risk factors for Alzheimer's disease are
    a. race, age
    b. age, family history
    c. sex, family history
    d. diet, age, family history

31. Alzheimer's disease is identified by
    a. a blood test
    b. documentation of behaviors and symptoms over time
    c. an x-ray of the skull
    d. all of these

32. The home health aide caring for an Alzheimer's client needs
    a. patience
    b. understanding of the symptoms
    c. to know the client cannot help his or her behavior
    d. all of these

33. If the client has difficulty walking, the aide can
    a. remove scatter rugs
    b. pick up small objects on the floor
    c. a and b
    d. none of these

34. One way to prevent the client from wandering is to
    a. keep the client locked in a room
    b. keep the front door locked
    c. tell the client that his or her behavior is inappropriate
    d. none of these

# Unit 23   Caring for the Client with Cancer

## SHORT ANSWER/FILL IN THE BLANKS ....................................

Complete the following sentences with the correct word or words.

1. An uncontrolled growth of abnormal cells is called _____.

2. Cancer cells steal _____ from surrounding cells and push _____ cells out of the way.

3. Cancer cells cause changes in the body, producing _____ and _____ of something wrong.

4. The seven warning signs of cancer are:

   a. _____

   b. _____

   c. _____

   d. _____

   e. _____

   f. _____

   g. _____

5. A substance or agent that produces cancer is called a _____.

6. The process in which some cancerous cells break away from the original tumor and move to other parts of the body is called _____.

7. When cancer is treated and does not reappear for 5 years, the cancer is considered _____.

8. Each day, more than _____ people die from cancer.

9. There are more than _____ types of cancer.

10. Rays aimed deep into the body to reach cancer cells and destroy them are called _____.

11. Side effects of radiation include _____, _____ _____, _____ of the area, and loss of _____.

12. Precautions the home health aide should take when caring for a client who has just had chemotherapy are:

    a. _____

    b. _____

    c. _____

13. The client with cancer needs to have a diet high in _____ and _____.

14. The client with cancer may have a distinctive _____ and may require a room _____.

15. The goal of cancer therapy in the final stages is to keep the client _____ and with the least amount of _____.

16. The dying client may be admitted to _____ care.

17. All women should have a yearly _____ to test for cancer of the _____.

18. If the female has cancer of the uterus, a _____ may be necessary.

19. After a mastectomy, the client needs to follow the _____ program started at the hospital; the home health aide can help the client with this.

20. A free service provided by the American Cancer Society available to the postmastectomy client is called _____ _____ _____ _____.

21. After mastectomy, a _____ may be made for the client.

22. Several illnesses affecting the respiratory system are _____, _____, and _____.

23. Five signs of lung cancer are:

    a. _____

    b. _____

    c. _____

    d. _____

    e. _____

24. Removal of part of the lung is called _____.

25. The client with lung cancer may require _____ therapy.

26. If the client has trouble breathing in the lying down position, many _____ should be offered.

27. The client may have a lot of secretions in the lungs, and the aide must use _____ _____ when handling these secretions.

28. The part of the trachea called the voice box is the _____.

29. A treatment for cancer of the larynx is removal of the larynx, or _____.

30. The trachea is the airway between the nasal passages and the _____.

31. A surgical opening into the trachea is called a _____.

32. The dressing over the tracheostomy stoma should be kept _____ to avoid inhaling dust.

33. Speech therapists work with the client after a _____ to help the client to learn to speak again.

34. The home health aide needs to be alert to any _____ or _____ _____ from the tracheostomy.

35. The body wastes are expelled through an _____ in the abdomen after surgical removal of the large intestine. These wastes are liquid and drain constantly; they are an _____ to the skin.

36. Ostomies sometimes have odors. The home health aide can suggest _____. It is important to be tactful in doing this because the client may feel _____.

37. Skin cancer is most often caused by excessive exposure to the _____.

## TRUE OR FALSE

Answer the following statements true (T) or false (F).

38. T   F   The exact cause of cancer is unknown.

39. T   F   Carcinogens can be chemical, environmental factors, hormones, or viruses.

40. T   F   Cancer is the leading cause of death each year.

41. T   F   A hysterectomy inhibits the enjoyment of sex for the woman.

42. T   F   Fibroid tumors of the uterus are not cancerous.

43. T   F   After hysterectomy, hormones are given to the female clients to replace those normally produced.

44. T   F   There has been an increase in cancer of the colon and stomach each year.

45. T   F   If a woman notices a lump in her breast, she can wait until her next regularly scheduled appointment to tell her physician.

46. T   F   Sometimes the physician will perform a lumpectomy instead of a mastectomy.

47. T   F   It is important for a woman to have the support of her family after undergoing a mastectomy.

48. T   F   Only lung cancer exceeds colon cancer in the number of new cases and deaths each year.

49. T   F   One treatment for cancer of the colon is a colostomy.

## MATCHING

Match each term with the proper definition.

50. _____ carcinogen
51. _____ malignant
52. _____ benign
53. _____ biopsy
54. _____ remission changes
55. _____ metastasis
56. _____ mammogram
57. _____ mastectomy
58. _____ hysterectomy
59. _____ chemotherapy

a. noncancerous
b. no longer growing
c. surgical removal of the uterus
d. use of chemicals to attack cancer
e. sample of tissue from the area with cellular changes
f. x-ray of breast
g. cancerous
h. cancer producing
i. surgical removal of breast
j. spreading of the cancer to other tissues

## DOCUMENTATION EXERCISES

60. You are caring for Mrs. Plum. She is recovering from a mastectomy. She is weeping and very upset. She is convinced that she is going to die, even though the physician has informed her that the tumor was very small and the chances of it recurring are very slight. Mrs. Plum's family is very supportive of her. How will you reassure her? What can you tell her relatives? Document your care.

_____

_____

61. You are assigned to care for Mr. Ken. He has just returned from the hospital, where he received a chemotherapy treatment. He feels very fatigued. He sometimes becomes nauseated after chemotherapy. What precautions do you need to take? He tells you that he is not hungry. What can you do to encourage Mr. Ken to eat?

_____

_____

## MULTIPLE CHOICE ········································································

Choose the correct answer or answers.

62. Diets for clients with cancer are usually
    a. low calorie
    b. semiliquid
    c. high calorie, high protein
    d. diabetic diets

63. It is important for women to perform breast self-examinations
    a. once a week
    b. once a year
    c. once a month
    d. only if they choose not to see a physician every year

64. Removal of the breast is called
    a. appendectomy
    b. mastectomy
    c. hysterectomy
    d. none of these

65. Signs of lung cancer include
    a. constant vomiting, earache
    b. high fever, coughing
    c. coughing up blood, chest pain
    d. none of these

# Unit 24  Caring for the Client with AIDS

## SHORT ANSWER/FILL IN THE BLANKS ··········································

Complete the following sentences with the correct word or words.

1. A severe immunological disorder caused by the human immunodeficiency virus is called _____ _____, or _____.

2. The HIV virus can be transmitted by intimate contact with body fluids in the _____, _____ or _____ _____ _____.

3. A disease transmitted by sexual intercourse is referred to as an _____.

4. It has been estimated that HIV has infected _____ to _____ million adults and _____ million children.

5. A client infected with AIDS can display many signs and symptoms; no two are _____.

6. Each client's care plan will need to be _____.

7. Infants can be infected by the mother's _____.

8. The incubation period for AIDS can be _____ to _____ _____.

9. It is important for the home health aide to know AIDS is a disease and the people who are infected require _____ just like any other ill person.

10. There is _____ _____ to prevent AIDS.

11. There is no _____ for AIDS.

12. The only way to control the disease is _____.

13. The home health aide should wear a _____ if there is a possibility of soiling clothes with body secretions. Wear gloves and wash hands before and after _____ _____; discard articles contaminated with body secretions or blood in a red biohazard container.

14. If the home health aide has an open cut or wound, it needs to be _____ before caring for an AIDS client.

15. The home health aide needs to follow _____ _____ with the AIDS client.

16. The home health aide _____ _____ _____ to friends, neighbors, or anyone else the nature of a client's illness.

17. A test for the AIDS virus can remain negative for up to _____ _____.

18. A client with AIDS sometimes reacts unstable emotionally; the aide needs to offer _____ _____.

19. If the client has diarrhea, the aide can offer _____ _____.

20. The main cleaning agent used in the home should be _____.

## TRUE OR FALSE

Answer the following statements true (T) or false (F).

21. T   F   AIDS cannot be transmitted by kissing, coughing, drinking from the same glasses, or sharing dishes.

22. T   F   In most cases, AIDS is transferred by sexual contact, drug users sharing needles, and babies infected before birth.

23. T   F   AIDS can be transmitted by blood transfusion.

24. T   F   The AIDS client should be educated about prevention of the transmission of the disease.

25. T   F   It is all right to give care to the AIDS client when the aide has open sores or wounds.

26. T   F   If the home health aide has a bad cold or other infection, the aide should not care for any clients.

27. T   F   The home health aide needs to become best friends with the client.

28. T   F   Allow your client to feel anger and frustration.

29. T   F   It is important to encourage the client to become involved in the care plan.

30. T   F   AIDS is a punishment from God for sinful sexual practices.

## DOCUMENTATION EXERCISES

31. You are caring for Mr. Jones, who has AIDS. You have been caring for him for several months. Today, you cannot seem to do anything to please him. He does not like the meal you prepared. He complains that the vacuum is too noisy. What do you do? What can you say to him to make him understand how you are feeling?

_____

_____

32. Your client, Mr. Jones, has vomited in the kitchen and you have to clean it up. What precautions will you take? What will you document?

_____

_____

## MULTIPLE CHOICE

Choose the correct answer or answers.

33. AIDS is transmitted by
   a. kissing
   b. sharing the same eating utensils
   c. sexual contact
   d. sleeping in the same bed

34. Symptoms of AIDS include
   a. diarrhea
   b. night sweats
   c. confusion
   d. all of these

35. Protection against AIDS includes
   a. practicing safe sex
   b. not sharing needles
   c. using gloves
   d. a and b only

36. The home health aide caring for the AIDS client who is experiencing diarrhea needs to
   a. encourage fluid intake
   b. use gloves
   c. record amount and frequency of stools
   d. all of these

# Unit 25   Maternal Care

## SHORT ANSWER/FILL IN THE BLANKS

Complete the following sentences with the correct word or words.

1. A woman should seek medical care when she thinks she might be _____.

2. Frequent urination is due to the enlarged _____ on the bladder.

3. The uterus dropping into the pelvic cavity signals a condition known as _____ .

4. One of the most common symptoms of pregnancy is _____, which may last up to 12 weeks.

5. Diminished gastric motility during pregnancy can cause _____.

6. Flatulence during pregnancy may be due to gas-forming _____ in the intestine.

7. Pressure exerted by the pregnant uterus on the intestines can cause _____.

8. Interference with circulation in the veins during pregnancy can lead to _____ and _____.

9. The pressure of the enlarging uterus on the diaphragm causes _____ _____, which will resolve when _____ occurs.

10. Many pregnant women experience backaches; wearing _____ shoes and practicing good _____ will help minimize this.

11. Leg cramps can also occur; _____ and frequent rest _____ with the feet _____ helps relieve this problem.

12. In the hot weather, _____ of the feet may occur.

13. High-risk pregnancies can cause low _____, premature, or brain damaged _____.

14. Down's syndrome generally occurs in women over the age of _____.

15. Prenatal tests, including _____, amniocentesis, and blood tests, are available to high-risk mothers.

16. Adolescent mothers do not always seek prenatal care because of _____, denial, or lack of _____.

17. A very serious complication that can occur during pregnancy when the mother drinks excessively is known as _____ _____ _____.

18. Examples of high-risk mothers include women who have had a history of spontaneous _____, _____ _____, or difficult pregnancies in the past.

19. Possible signs of miscarriage include _____ associated with abdominal _____ and severe abdominal _____ and bleeding.

20. Danger signals include persistent _____, chills, _____, sudden escape of _____ from the vaginal area, swelling of the face or finger, and severe headache. If the home health aide notices these signals, the aide needs to _____ _____.

21. Home health aide care for the pregnant woman generally is necessary only if the mother is _____ _____.

22. Five things the home health aide needs to remember when caring for a pregnant client are:

a. _____

b. _____

c. _____

d. _____

e. _____

23. Lochia is the bloody vaginal discharge following the normal _____.

24. Lochia should not have a foul _____.

25. Breast _____ is painful. The aide can offer _____ _____ and suggest that the client wear a _____ _____.

26. The perineal incision made during delivery is called an _____.

27. Pain from incisions can be helped by the use of a _____ _____.

28. As the uterus contracts during the postpartum period, the client will have _____. This can be relieved by medication prescribed by the physician.

29. The new mother may experience difficulty in _____ for about 24 hours.

## TRUE OR FALSE

Answer the following statements true (T) or false (F).

30. T F Fetal alcohol syndrome causes babies to be underweight and mentally deficient.

31. T F Deficiencies in the diet of the mother can result in low birthweight babies.

32. T F Tobacco use during pregnancy generally does not harm the baby.

33. T F Drug-addicted babies can result from drug-addicted mothers.

34. T F The home health aide should encourage the pregnant mother to be optimistic.

35. T F The postpartum period is defined as that period preceding the birth of the child.

36. T F Breast engorgement occurs immediately after delivery.

37. T F The new mother may find that she is sweating more than usual. This is normal.

38. T F Postpartum blues are relatively rare.

39. T F The new mother needs to rest as much as she can.

## DOCUMENTATION EXERCISES

40. You are caring for a new mother. She has three other children under the age of 5. You are to care for the family as well as the new mother. The younger children are constantly wanting to bother their mother. What can you do to let Mrs. Pal get some well-deserved rest? Document your response.

_____

_____

41. Your client, Mrs. Dell is breast-feeding her newborn. Mrs. Dell's mother is visiting. She tells Mrs. Dell that the baby is not getting enough milk and that is why the baby cries a lot. You know that all babies and mothers need a time to adjust to each other. What can you do to help the situation. What will you say to Mrs. Dell's mother?

_____

_____

## MULTIPLE CHOICE

Choose the correct answer or answers.

42. Discomforts of pregnancy include
    a. nausea, constipation, heartburn
    b. coughing, temperature
    c. loose stools, high temperature
    d. chest pain, difficult breathing

43. New mothers are released from hospitals after
    a. 1 week
    b. 3 days
    c. 24 to 48 hours
    d. after 6 days

44. The home health aide caring for a new mother at home should watch for and report to the case manager immediately if the client
   a. is weeping and feeling blue
   b. has bright red vaginal bleeding
   c. has headache and tiredness
   d. all of these

# Unit 26   Infant Care

## SHORT ANSWER/FILL IN THE BLANKS

Complete the following sentences with the correct word or words.

1. The birth of a baby is an _____ for both parents and child.

2. The individuals who meet the infant's primary needs influence its _____ and _____ _____.

3. Feeding the infant should be an _____, _____ time.

4. Breast milk is the _____ food for any infant.

5. Bottle-feeding allows members of the family to _____ in feeding the infant.

6. The baby should be placed on his or her stomach only if _____, _____ _____ _____, or _____ _____.

7. The baby should be burped after drinking _____ to _____ ounces of formula or between breasts.

8. If the baby is circumcised, the penis should be _____ and covered with _____ each time the diaper is changed.

9. The redness and the secretions from the circumcision should disappear within _____ _____.

10. The uncircumcised infant's penis should be cleansed with _____ and _____.

## TRUE OR FALSE

Answer the following statements true (T) or false (F).

11. T   F   Physical and emotional well-being are intimately related to each other.

12. T   F   Caring for a newborn baby comes naturally to new parents.

13. T   F   Newborn infants will triple their birthweight in 1 year.

14. T   F   The baby should be placed on the stomach.

## DOCUMENTATION EXERCISES

15. You are caring for an infant, Bobby. He is only 3 days old. Every time you feed him, he vomits. His mother says he has been throwing up since he was born. She has tried two different formulas, but he still vomits. What would you do? Who would you contact? How would you document this?

_____

_____

16. You are caring for twins. Their mother had cesarean surgery, and you are her helper. You are assigned to bathe the infants and assist the mother with bathing. You are also assigned to prepare meals and launder clothes. Document your care.

_____

_____

## MULTIPLE CHOICE

Choose the correct answer or answers.

17. When bottle feeding an infant, you need to
    a. prop the bottle
    b. burp the baby after every 2 to 3 ounces of fluid
    c. place the baby on the stomach after feeding is completed
    d. none of these

18. It is necessary to burp the baby to
    a. prevent the baby from overeating
    b. give the baby a rest from eating
    c. allow removal of air the baby swallowed while eating
    d. all of these

19. Breast milk is the best milk for the baby because
    a. the major ingredients are suited to the infants needs
    b. the milk will not be spoiled
    c. the mother will cuddle the baby while feeding
    d. all of these

20. The infant should be given a sponge bath
    a. until the stump of the umbilical cord falls off          c. twice a day
    b. to conserve water                                         d. none of these

21. When the home health aide is bathing the infant, the aide should
    a. notice the skin condition                                 c. relax and talk softly to the infant
    b. make sure all the soap is rinsed off the infant          d. all of these

# Unit 27   Job-Seeking Skills

## SHORT ANSWER/FILL IN THE BLANKS

Complete the following sentences with the correct word or words.

1. The need for home health services has increased in the past _____ _____.

2. Three places to look for employment are:

    a. _____

    b. _____

    c. _____

3. When going to the interview, it is better to go _____.

4. You should dress _____ and _____ _____ _____ for the interview.

5. It is a good idea to arrive at the interview _____.

6. Bring with you to the interview all papers that will be required. This may include _____ _____, _____, and _____ _____ _____.

7. After the interview, send a thank you _____.

8. Generally personal references should not include _____.

9. Take care to fill out the application _____ and to follow the instructions exactly.

10. Many states have mandatory requirements for hiring _____ _____ _____.

## MULTIPLE CHOICE

Choose the correct answer or answers.

11. When the home health aide prepares for the interview, he or she needs to
    a. dress neatly
    b. have clean, neatly styled hair
    c. make eye contact with the interviewer
    d. all of these

12. It is important to find out information about a job before accepting it. Some of the information the home health aide needs to consider is
    a. the travel distance required
    b. the benefits, including insurance and holidays
    c. the number of hours of work required
    d. all of these

## DOCUMENTATION EXERCISES

13. You accept employment with a home health agency. When you arrive at the home to be oriented, the case manager tells you that you will be responsible for a 2-week-old infant. You specified on your employment application that you did not feel comfortable caring for newborns. How will you handle this situation? They are counting on you to care for the mother and the infant.

_____

_____

14. You have misplaced your social security card. You are scheduled for an appointment to be interviewed in 1 hour. How will you handle this situation?

_____

_____

15. You have been employed by a home health agency. You go in to receive your assignment and discover the location of the client is 50 miles from the office. You explained to the interviewer at orientation that you would not be able to travel more than a few miles because your car was not functioning well. The nurse orienting you told you this would not be a problem. What can you do?

_____

_____

16. You arrive 20 minutes early for your job interview. You look for a parking place, but none is available near the location of the agency. Finally, you find a parking place 8 blocks from the agency location. You will never make it on time. What could you have done to prevent this situation?

_____

_____

17. Fill out the practice application for employment, Figure 27-1.

CUSHMAN MANAGEMENT ASSOCIATES

APPLICATION FOR EMPLOYMENT

We are an equal opportunity employer. Federal and state laws prohibit discrimination in employment policies based on race, color, religion, sex, age, handicap, disability, or national origin. No question on this
application is asked for the purpose of limiting or excluding any applicant's consideration for employment
because of his or her race, color, religion, sex, age, handicap, disability, or national origin.

| Name:   Last         First         Middle | Social Security No. | Telephone No. |
|---|---|---|

| Address:   Street   City   State   Zip Code | Licensed Nurses Only | |
|---|---|---|
| | Mass. Reg. No. | Date Granted: |

| If your records may be under a name other than indicated above, please specify: | Last Renewal: | Expiration Date: |
|---|---|---|

| Are you a citizen of the United States?  ☐ yes  ☐ no | If you are not a U.S. Citizen, do you have the legal right to remain permanently in the United States?  ☐ yes  ☐ no | Explain |
|---|---|---|
| Are you between the ages of 18 and 70?  ☐ yes  ☐ no | Do you know of any fact that would limit or impair your ability to perform the functions of the job you are applying for?  ☐ yes  ☐ no | Describe |

| Date of last Physical Examination: | Family Physician: | I authorize my doctor to release to you the results of my pre-employment and subsequent medical examinations, and to discuss those results with you.  ☐ yes  ☐ no |
|---|---|---|

| Position desired: | Hours desired: | Salary expected: |
|---|---|---|

Specialized training or experience
not shown on other side of form:

| Where now employed? | Reason for desiring change: |
|---|---|

Have you ever pleaded guilty  ☐ yes        If yes to either, please explain:
or been convicted of a felony?  ☐ no

or a misdemeanor other than a first conviction
for drunkenness, simple assault, speeding, minor        ☐ yes
traffic violations, affray, or disturbance of the peace  ☐ no
within the past 5 years?

| In case of emergency notify | name                    relationship |
|---|---|
| | address                   telephone |

\* I authorize the schools, employers, and individuals listed in this application to release any information regarding my previous employment,
character, general reputation and personal characteristics.     ☐ yes   ☐ no

I certify that the statements I have made in this application are true and hereby grant the employer permission to verify the accuracy and completeness of this
information and to investigate all references and educational records. I understand that any false or misleading statements made by me on this application or in
conjunction with my physical examination will be sufficient cause for the rejection of this application or for immediate dismissal if such false or misleading
information is discovered after my employment. If I am accepted for employment, I agree to abide by the rules and regulations of the employer.

Signed _____

Date _____

"It is unlawful in Massachusetts to require or administer a lie detector test as a condition of employment or continued employment. An employer who violates this
law shall be subject to criminal penalties and civil liability."

**FIGURE 27-1**

## TO THE EMPLOYEE

Because you are important to us, we want to help you develop a good work record. If we feel that you are violating any of our rules and policies, or that you have misunderstood the terms of employment, we will hold a conference with you. Continued *infractions* will cause your immediate dismissal. PLEASE READ THE FOLLOWING CAREFULLY.

1. *Attendance and tardiness record:* Recurring cancellations of promised scheduled workdays may result in dismissal. Absence without call in may result in immediate termination. No pay raises will be granted if attendance and tardiness records are unsatisfactory. We must be able to depend on you. You must call in if you are unable to meet your assignment.

2. *Unbecoming conduct:* Any of the following are considered to be gross *misconduct:* carelessness and inattention to client care; failure to perform duties; violation of safe practices; inefficiency and wasting of materials; refusal to obey direct orders; insubordination; rude, discourteous or uncivil behavior; intoxication, drinking, or possession of intoxicating beverages while on duty; gambling on duty; sleeping on duty; unauthorized absence from assignment or leaving early without permission; failure to report an injury or accident concerning an employee or client; soliciting tips from clients or families; sale of services to clients or families; divulging confidential information about client and family; theft and/or dishonesty; *pilferage* of drugs or violation of any law on drug use including use or sale of same; damaging, defacing or mishandling equipment or property; interfering with work performance of another employee; falsifying client or personnel records or any form of misrepresentation.

Employee's statement:

I have read the above rules and regulations and understand my responsibilities to the agency and client. I agree to abide by these terms of employment.

_____     _____
Employee Signature                                                              Date

_____     _____
Supervisor's Signature                                                          Date

**FIGURE 27-1**

# SECTION THREE
# Crossword Puzzles

# Unit 1

## Across

2. the learning behavior patterns of a race, nation, or people
4. usually in the home; keeps the client company
5. assesses the client's ability to communicate, understand, and write; works to rehabilitate the client
7. member of the health care team who coordinates all the services the client may require
8. begins suddenly and is usually severe
9. group that cares for dying clients and their families

## Down

1. performs personal and nursing care skills
3. assesses the client's condition and determines the type of personal and nursing care needed; provides care
4. lasts a long time
6. final life-ending stage
10. Omnibus Budget Reconciliation Act

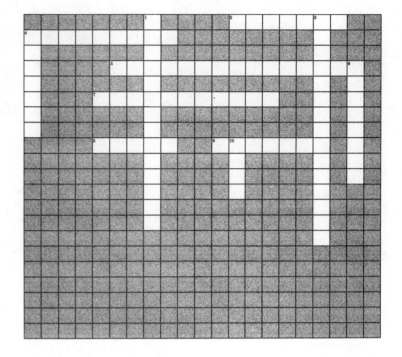

# Unit 2

## Across

1. personal cleanliness of the human body
5. to record on proper form your observations and actions
6. treatment that reasonably could cause physical pain, mental anguish, or fear
7. the practical and necessary information one must learn about a subject
8. gathering information about changes in the client's conditions or behavior, using your five senses

## Down

2. the reciprocating actions between two people or between members of a group
3. the separate parts of a machine or a procedure that make up the whole
4. to make a written record or oral summary of the care of a client

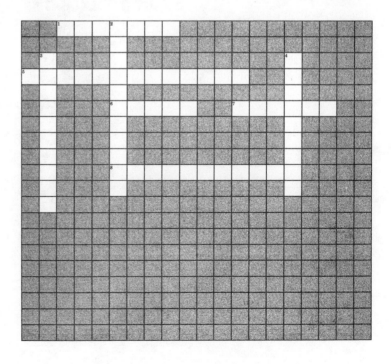

# Unit 3

## Across

1. the sending and receiving of messages, may be verbal or nonverbal
3. without placing value judgment on the actions or words of others
4. a form of communication using gestures and facial expressions instead of words
5. restating in your own words what the other person has said
6. paraphrasing the other person's words using your own words
7. hearing with thoughtful attention
8. communicating without words using gestures, expressions, or body movement

## Down

2. listening to the speaker, reflecting the speaker's feelings, and commenting on them to the speaker
5. offering reassurances that are not valid to another person

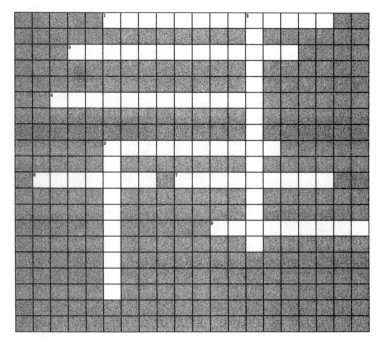

# Unit 4

## Across

1. gait belt
6. away from the center
8. to hold rigidly in one position
9. to turn
11. lack of oxygen in the blood causing the client to appear bluish

## Down

2. to work together
3. the technique used to get the most effective and least taxing body movements
4. to empty or remove the contents of
5. technique for removing a food particle or foreign object lodged in the trachea
7. belt used to assist client movements
10. that which is dangerous or could cause a serious accident

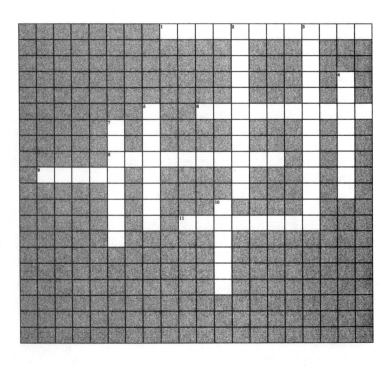

# Unit 5

### Across

7. microorganisms causing disease
8. roughage foods needed by the body to prevent constipation and to keep stool soft
9. a specialty store selling cheeses, cold cuts, sodas, sandwiches, and convenience foods
10. a fuzzy, gray fungus growth that appears in damp, dark areas

### Down

1. those foodstuffs that are the basis for preparing foods and normally kept in most homes
2. the steps taken to accomplish a particular task
3. of or relating to health and cleanliness
4. fabric that requires no ironing
5. an inborn trait
6. likely to spoil or decay

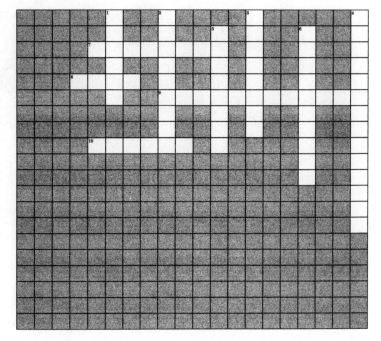

# Unit 6

### Across

2. condition when there is impaired muscular power and coordination because of a lack of oxygen to the brain
5. sudden infant death syndrome
7. the time required from conception to birth
8. unborn child
10. the ability to resist certain diseases
11. the period of physical and emotional development from early teens to young adulthood
13. a process of attachment of mother, father, and infant happening immediately after birth
14. an infant born before full term

### Down

1. occurs when a female egg is fertilized by a male sperm
2. an inherited condition that affects children's sweat glands, pancreas, and respiratory system
3. a full-term baby weighing less than 5 pounds
4. brothers and sisters
6. sexually transmitted diseases
9. the time period following childhood when the body matures and reproduction becomes possible
12. emotional or physical abuse of an individual under the age of 18

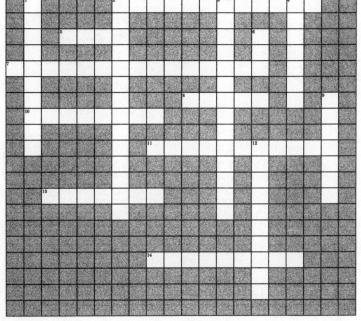

# Unit 7

*Across*

7. period between 25 and 45 years of age
9. direct examination of the interior of the sigmoid colon
10. a progressive disease involving the nerves of the brain and the spinal cord

*Down*

1. the probable outcome of an illness
2. to avoid illness before it starts
3. value one places on one's self as a person functioning in society
4. period between 45 and 65 years of age
5. cessation of the monthly menstrual cycle
6. x-rays of the female breasts used to determine whether a tumor is present
8. a medical technique whereby a sample of the vaginal cells are tested for cancer

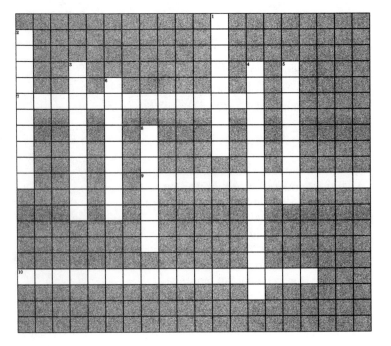

# Unit 8

*Across*

4. loss of bone density and strength
7. starchy foods

*Down*

1. loss of voluntary control of bladder muscles, causing uncontrolled voiding
2. progressive mental deterioration caused by organic brain disease
3. severance of something
5. a mental state characterized by loss of hope, feelings of rejection, and generalized sadness
6. usually refers to persons over the age of 65

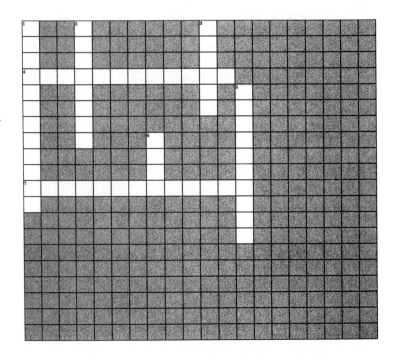

# Unit 9

*Across*

2. contains pathogens that may lead to infection
5. lung disease
7. procedure whereby client is kept away from others to prevent spread of a contagious disease
8. microorganisms capable of causing disease
9. microorganisms that can cause disease and live on lice, ticks, fleas, and mites
11. inflammation of the liver
13. microorganisms causing disease
14. technique to rid the environment of microorganisms and provide a sterile area
17. tiny one-celled animals
18. yellowish color of skin, eyes, and mucous membranes
19. microorganism that lives and grows by feeding on living cells

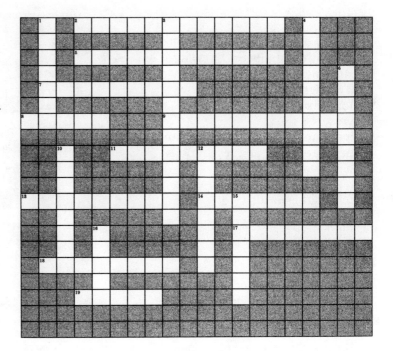

*Down*

1. free of pathogens
3. organisms not visible to the naked eye that can cause disease
4. diseases that can spread from one person to another
6. invasion of pathogenic organisms causing infection
10. one-celled microorganisms
12. hostile entry into another area or place
15. ability to observe and share feelings of others in a supportive manner
16. microorganisms that cause vaginitis and athlete's foot

# Unit 10

*Across*

4. permanent shortening of muscle tissue causing deformity or distortion
5. slow pulse
6. a change that can be observed
7. force exerted by blood on walls of blood vessels
10. measurements of blood pressure, temperature, pulse, and respirations
12. heartbeats per minute
13. measurement of blood pressure when the heart is beating
14. lasts a long time
16. difficult or labored respirations

*Down*

1. restoring mental and physical abilities after an accident or illness
2. absence of breathing
3. one of the vital signs in which the breaths of a person are counted
4. respiration characterized by periods of apnea and periods of dyspnea
8. blood pressure measurement when heart is relaxing
9. those changes reported by the client
11. begins suddenly and is usually severe
15. bubbling sound from lungs when mucus or fluid is trapped in air passages

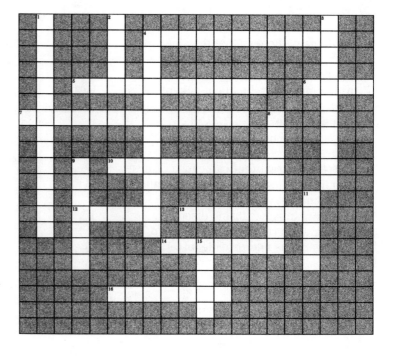

# Units 11 and 12

*Across*

2. mental state characterized by loss of hope, feelings of rejection, and generalized sadness
4. drug used to reduce fluid accumulation in the body
5. a condition resulting from poor diet that lacks needed nutrients
8. changes a person makes in behavior to adjust to a situation
10. sum of those processes using food for growth, development, and body maintenance
11. food prepared without spices and consisting of easily digested food
12. progressive mental deterioration caused by organic brain disease
13. basic feelings common to all (fear, love, anger, sorrow, and anxiety)

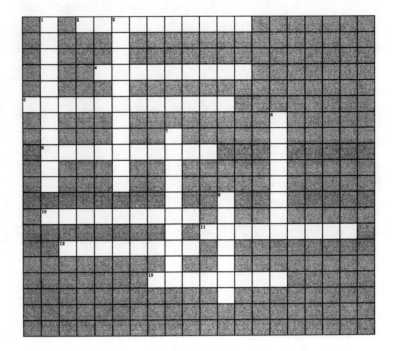

*Down*

1. one who does not eat meat or meat products
3. involuntary wavelike movements that move food through the digestive tract
7. process by which the body burns fuel
6. feces lodged in the intestine
9. a measure of energy

# Unit 13

*Across*

3. mucous-lined tube conveying urine from the bladder to the exterior of the body
4. inflammation of the bladder
6. process of introducing fluid into the rectum to remove feces and flatus
8. plastic or rubber placed into the body to release fluids
10. primary organ of the urinary system
11. infrequent or difficult bowel movements with hard feces
12. opening into

*Down*

1. muscular organ for storing urine
2. surgically formed opening between a body cavity or passage and the body's surface
5. loss of voluntary control of bladder muscles, causing uncontrolled voiding
7. medication used to stimulate bowels to eliminate feces
9. tube connecting the kidney to the bladder through which urine flows into the bladder

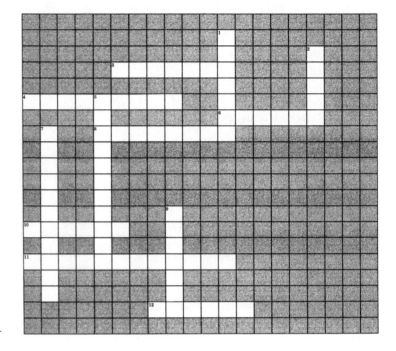

# Units 14 and 15

*Across*

1. degenerative bone disease of the cartilage
4. condition that exists when body temperature falls below 95°F
6. bed sore or dermal ulcer
7. condition causing tissues or organs to weaken
11. form of arthritis caused by an increased amount of uric acid in the diet
12. area between anus and vagina on females, and the scrotum in males
13. break in a bone
14. inner layer of skin

*Down*

2. medication that relieves inflammation
3. outer layer of skin
4. heatstroke
5. autoimmune response that results in inflammation of the joints
8. tough fibers holding bones in place
9. inflammation of a joint
10. hormonal medications used to treat many conditions

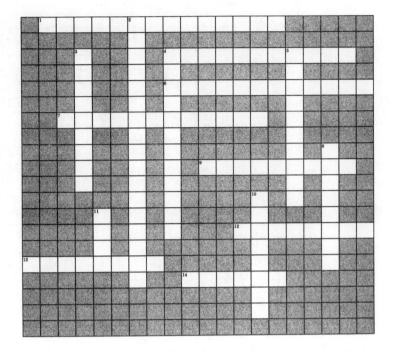

# Units 16–18

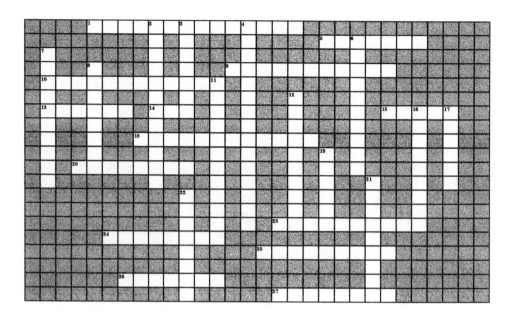

## Across

1. drug that prevents clot formation in the blood
5. a floating blood clot
9. having to do with breathing
10. chronic, progressive deafness, especially to low tones
13. disorder of respiratory system characterized by wheezing, coughing, and labored breathing
14. stroke
15. water retention, causing swelling of legs, arms, or other body part
18. paralysis of the four extremities
20. formation of large areas of dead tissue
23. paralysis of lower body involving both legs
24. pertaining to the ear or hearing
25. inflammation of the lungs
26. convulsion
27. localized enlargement of a blood vessel

## Down

2. permanent shortening of muscle tissue, causing deformity
3. difficulty speaking
4. fatty tissue collected within a blood vessel, causing impairment
6. inflammation on the bronchi
7. heart muscle
8. lack of blood supply
11. under the tongue
12. weakness or paralysis confined to one side of the body
16. condition of lung tissue where elastic characteristics have been lost
17. blood vessel carrying oxygenated blood to the tissues
19. chest pain
21. inflammation of vein
22. blood clot that forms inside an artery

# Units 19 and 20

*Across*

3. refers to a type of diabetes
8. bluish skin tone
12. product of body glands that assists in healthy body function
14. high blood sugar
16. sloughing off of the uterine lining of nonpregnant females
17. imbalanced acid base in body caused by loss of salts, sodium, and potassium
18. saclike organ containing testes

*Down*

1. chronic disorder related to metabolism
2. female hormone
3. instrument used to measure levels of blood sugar
4. male hormone
5. any disease of the nerves
6. painful menstruation
7. hormone produced by the islets of Langerhans
9. low blood sugar
10. sexually transmitted virus
11. venereal disease
13. a sexually transmitted disease usually starting with an ulcer
15. mouth of the uterus

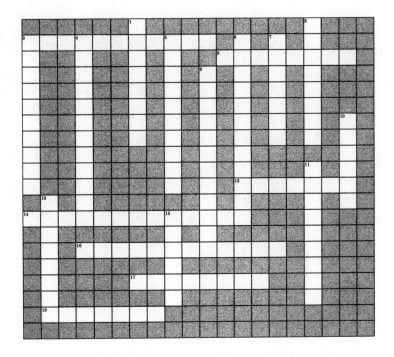

# Units 21–26

*Across*

1. techniques used to make people feel good about themselves
7. life-ending stage
9. a substance or agent that produces cancer
11. treatment for cancer in which chemicals are used to destroy the cancerous cells
13. feeling of separation or loss
15. gas or air in the intestine expelled from a body opening
16. a progressively degenerative illness that causes loss of memory and mental capacity
19. after death
23. removal of the uterus
24. removing part of the colon and making an opening on the abdomen
27. x-rays of the female breast
28. partial removal of a lung
29. the voice box
31. microscopic examination of a sample of tissue
32. group that provides specialized care for dying clients and their relatives
33. vaginal discharge after childbirth

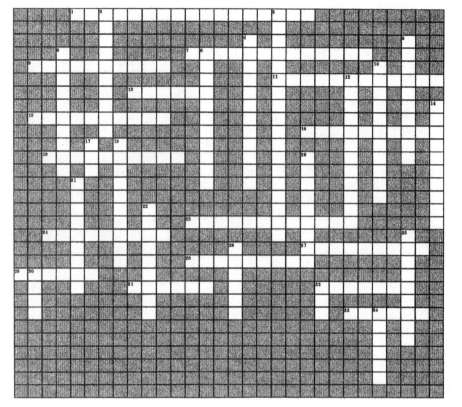

*Down*

2. legal document outlining medical care desired if a person cannot make independent decisions
3. documents specifying type of treatment individuals desire under serious medical conditions
4. removal of foreskin from penis
5. time during birth when baby's head settles into the pelvis before birth
6. use of fluid to cleanse area
8. to spit
10. talking about events that occurred earlier in life
12. an opening in the trachea
14. surgical removal of the female breast
17. sexually transmitted disease
18. time period after birth
20. removal of diseased small intestine and use of external abdominal stoma for removal of liquid stool
21. removing blood and fluid from a dead body and replacing with chemical preservative
22. period of illness when symptoms cease or become less severe
25. moving about without specific purpose
30. acquired immunodeficiency syndrome
32. human immunodeficiency virus
34. a disease characterized by rapid growth of abnormal cells
36. noncancerous

# Unit 27

### *Across*

2. carelessness in attention to client care, failure to perform duties, violation of safe practices
5. jobs available in a community
6. not a relative, but can include ministers, physicians, and instructors who had contact with applicant

### *Down*

1. services that obtain jobs in an area and send applicants to interviews
3. acronym for system of reimbursing hospitals, which controls costs
4. violation of company rules and policies

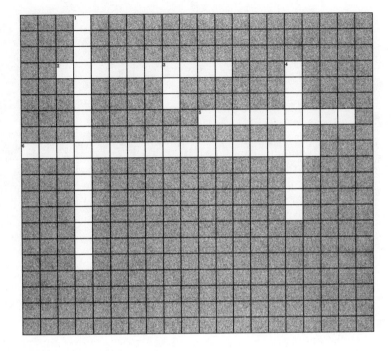

# SECTION FOUR
# Quizzes

# Quiz A

Answer the following statements true (T) or false (F).

1. T   F   If you are unsure of the correct terminology to use on the medical record, you should notify your case manager and ask for assistance.

2. T   F   You seem to be having a difficult time getting to know your client and are hesitant to do things for him. You should report this to your case manager.

3. T   F   The client insists that you give her a tub bath, even though the plan of care states that she should have a sponge bath. This should be reported to the agency before the change is made.

4. T   F   Mrs. Doe states that she does not feel like eating the breakfast you have prepared. Your documentation should state that client is a picky eater.

5. T   F   You should always document fact.

6. T   F   Clients may not read their medical records.

7. T   F   Subjective reporting means that you did not actually see something, but it was told to you.

8. T   F   You accidentally break a coffee cup belonging to your client. There is no need to fill out an accident report.

9. T   F   You see that it is getting much more difficult to transfer the client into the bathtub. This should be reported to your case manager.

10. T   F   While you are at your agency, you tell anyone who will listen to you how your client's daughter was in trouble with the law. This is acting in an ethical manner.

# Quiz B

Answer the following statements true (T) or false (F).

1. T   F   A homemaker/home health aide needs orientation to the client and the plan of care.

2. T   F   One of the duties of a homemaker/home health aide is to give insulin to the client when the family member is unable.

3. T   F   Anyone of any age can give home care with little or no training as long as the individual is comfortable with the job.

4. T   F   One of the services a client might receive is speech therapy.

5. T   F   When you find a home situation unsafe, you should correct the situation without any discussion with the case manager.

6. T   F   If you are going to be delayed in reaching the client's home, you should notify the agency.

7. T   F   When a family member asks you to do something you are unable to do, you should try to complete the service as best you can.

8. T F You may give the client an aspirin from your personal supply.

9. T F Simple meal preparation may need to be done for some clients.

10. T F You should notify the case manager if a family member states that the client no longer needs home care.

11. T F You might see two or more clients in 1 day.

12. T F The client's personal belongings need to be treated carefully and with respect.

# Quiz C

Answer the following statements true (T) or false (F).

1. T F A chronic illness is sudden and does not last very long.

2. T F Many individuals with disabilities will be able to tell you what you need to do for them.

3. T F It is okay to do everything for clients while you are there because it would take forever to let them do it for themselves.

4. T F Defense mechanisms, such as withdrawal and anger, are harmful to the client who uses these all the time.

5. T F Chemical dependency is a disease that can be treated.

6. T F Mentally retarded individuals cannot learn to read.

7. T F Acute illness comes on suddenly and has a short duration.

8. T F People with physical disabilities may display periods of hopelessness.

9. T F People with mental illness are not really ill.

10. T F You may not always be able to meet all the needs of the mentally ill person.

# Quiz D

Answer the following statements true (T) or false (F).

1. T F It is permissible to smoke in your client's home when you need to be there for more than 4 hours.

2. T F A family member asks you to lend them some money because "things are tight right now." You are permitted to do this.

3. T F It is important for you as a homemaker/home health aide to present a positive attitude toward the client and the family.

4. T F You saw a visiting neighbor take something from your client's jewelry box. You need not call your case manager because this is none of your business.

5. T   F   You are asked by one of the family members to stay longer with the client. You should call your case manager.

# Quiz E

Complete the following sentences with the correct word or words.

1. A _____ or _____ is a nurse who is licensed by the state to practice.

2. An _____ _____ is a long-term problem.

3. A _____ _____ _____ is a facility for just the elderly patient.

4. A _____ _____ _____ _____ works with the client the most.

5. _____ are studies done to determine the numbers of days of hospitalization necessary for certain medical conditions.

# Quiz F

Complete the following sentences with the correct word or words.

1. A _____ _____ way of communication is to touch your client's hand gently.

2. The abbreviation tid means _____ _____ _____.

3. The use of special words and abbreviations in health care is called _____ _____.

# Quiz G

Match each term with the proper definition.

1. _____ expressive quality of voice that gives meaning
2. _____ communication without words
3. _____ sending and receiving of information
4. _____ inability to speak or use words correctly
5. _____ highness or lowness of a voice
6. _____ a feeling of anger
7. _____ a smile, frown, or arm motion
8. _____ complete lack of interest
9. _____ a syllable or word that appears at the beginning of a term
10. _____ a syllable or word that appears at the end of a term

a. body language
b. communication
c. tone
d. pitch
e. nonverbal expression
f. hostility
g. apathy
h. aphasia
i. suffix
j. prefix
k. dysphagia

# Quiz H

Choose the correct answer or answers.

1. Who plays an important role in giving emotional support to a client?
   a. clergy
   b. family members
   c. friends
   d. members of the home care team
   e. b and c
   f. a and b
   g. d only
   h. all of these

2. When illness strikes a family, it can cause
   a. anxiety
   b. worry
   c. financial loss
   d. all of these

3. When a client seems to be very apathetic about his or her plan of care, you should
   a. assume he or she is ill
   b. forget about it
   c. notify your case manager
   d. tell a family member

4. A person who is confined to bed for long periods can develop
   a. contractures
   b. atrophy
   c. constipation
   d. all of these

5. Alzheimer's disease affects people
   a. 16 to 24 years old
   b. who are mentally ill
   c. generally between 40 and 70 years of age
   d. who are injured by a blow to the head

# SECTION FIVE
# Case Studies

# Unit 1   Home Health Services

Read the following case studies and answer the questions.

## Case 1

Your neighbor requests information from you about home health care. She wants to know what it is.

### Questions

1. How do you get home health care?
2. Do home health agencies have to be licensed?
3. What can she do to work in home health?
4. She used to take care of her father before he died. What can you tell her?

## Case 2

You have worked for 10 years in a nursing home as a certified nurse's aide. Your employer goes out of business. Someone tells you about home health.

### Questions

1. What would have you do to find out more about home health?
2. What certification would you need?
3. Do you need to go to school?

# Unit 2   Responsibilities of the Home Health Aide

## Case 1

You are assigned to care for Mr. Lopez. When you arrive at Mr. Lopez's home, you are greeted by his daughter. She tells you that you are to make sure he takes his bath. When you enter Mr. Lopez's room to prepare for his bath, he tells you he is not taking a bath. You are aware that the client has the right to refuse care.

### Questions

1. What will you do?
2. What will you tell his daughter?
3. Do you need to contact your case manager?

## Case 2

While you are caring for Mr. Lopez, he urinates on the floor. He has not been incontinent before. While you are cleaning up the accident, he informs you not to tell anyone, in particular his daughter. Mr. Lopez tells you his daughter will put him in a nursing home if she finds out.

### Questions

1. What is the right thing to do?
2. You are expected to inform your case manager. Can you do this without telling Mr. Lopez?
3. What about Mr. Lopez's daughter, are you obligated to tell her?

# Unit 3   Developing Effective Communication Skills

## Case 1

You arrive at your client's house. Mr. Long looks very sad. You ask him what is wrong. He tells you that his dog has been hit by a car and is dead. He states "Spot was the only person left that loved me. Now I am all alone."

### Questions

1. What will you say to him?
2. Can you think of anything to cheer him up?

## Case 2

You are assigned to care for Mrs. Kay. She requires a bath, meal preparation, and laundry to be washed. When you arrive, her daughter is there with three children, all in diapers. She immediately starts telling you what she requires you to do. Feed her children, wash the laundry that she brought, and clean the kitchen. You know that you are being paid by Medicare to care only for your client, Mrs. Kay. Mrs. Kay is frightened and cannot explain your role to her daughter.

### Questions

1. How will you make sure your client is cared for and not intimidated by her daughter?
2. What will you do about all the expectations of Mrs. Kay's daughter?

## Case 3

When you explain to Mrs. Kay's daughter that you are being paid by Medicare to care for her mother, she informs you that all of the other home health aides do as she asks.

### Questions

1. What is your ethical obligation regarding this information?

# Unit 4   Safety

## Case 1

You arrive at your new client's home. Mr. Jaffe is sitting in the living room. Walking around the room are three chickens. From the looks of the house, they have been living there for some time. When you tell Mr. Jaffe that the chickens are causing a health hazard, he gets very upset and refuses to allow you to put them outside.

### Questions

1. What will you do?
2. How can you give good care to your client and not have him become angry at you?
3. Should you call your supervisor?

## Case 2

You are assigned to care for Mrs. Pack. She lives in a rural area. After you introduce yourself to her and explain to her what you will be doing, you go to the bathroom to prepare for bathing her. When you are looking around the house, you realize that there is no bathroom. You ask Mrs. Pack where the bathroom is. She informs you there is an outhouse out back and a water pump on the side of the house.

### Questions

1. What can you do to care properly for your client?
2. How can you avoid making her feel that you are looking down on her?
3. How will you warm the water?
4. Is an outhouse sanitary?

# Unit 5   Homemaking Service

## Case 1

You have been assigned to perform housekeeping chores at Mr. Santos's house. As you prepare to start cleaning, you notice cockroaches all over the kitchen. They are in the pantry, in the stove, and crawling on the cabinets. You had no idea that you would be asked to care for a mess like this.

### Questions

1. What would you do first?
2. What area would you start to work in?

## Case 2

You are cleaning house and preparing a meal for Mrs. Kay. You have 4 hours and you need to clean the kitchen, wash the laundry, change the bed linens, clean the bathroom, and take Mrs. Kay for a walk. You also are aware that Mrs. Kay has severe arthritis and moves very slowly.

### Questions

1. How will you organize your time?
2. In what order will you perform these tasks?

# Unit 6   Infancy to Adolescence

## Case 1

You are carrying for three children: Kathy, age 8; Johnny, age 6; and Judy, age 4. While you are bathing them, you notice on several large bruises on Kathy. You ask her what happened to cause these bruises? Kathy looks down and says "I fell." You are very concerned about this.

### Questions

1. What would you do?
2. Would you talk to the other children?
3. Would you talk to the parents?
4. What are your responsibilities as a home health aide?

## Case 2

When you are caring for you client, Mr. Thyme, you hear loud talking in the back bedroom. You go to the room and you hear Mr. Thyme's grandson and his friends. It sounds like they are taking drugs.

### Questions

1. What can you do?
2. Can you go into the room?
3. Should you talk to Mr. Thyme about your concerns?
4. If they are using illegal drugs, what must you do?

# Unit 7   Early and Middle Adulthood

## Case 1

You wake up an hour later than usual. You do not know why your alarm clock did not go off at the proper time. You realize that you are going to be late to care for Mr. Howe. This causes you to be become very anxious. Mr. Howe is a very particular client. He is recovering from a broken leg. He is an executive and worries all the time about schedules. He is angry that he is ill because it interferes with his work schedule. You call him and tell him you are running late. He grumbles but tells you to hurry up, he has a business client coming to his home to do business in about 2 hours.

### Questions

1. What will you do to give good care without rushing?
2. Will you be able to carry out your duties?

## Case 2

You are caring for Mrs. Lemmon. She is diabetic and has very poor eyesight. A car is in her driveway. She tells you that she drives to the store at least twice a week. You ask her how she can see to drive. She tells you she has been driving to the same store for more than 30 years and the car knows where to go.

### Questions

1. Can you inform your case manager?
2. What can you do about this situation?

3. You know that no matter what you say or do, as long as that car is there and she has the keys, she will drive it. What legal responsibility do you have?

# Unit 8   Older Adulthood

## Case 1

Mrs. Klein is your client. She is very sweet and very cooperative except in one area. She is constantly dribbling urine. You have asked her to wear diapers, but she refuses. She is unsteady on her feet, and you are worried about her falling by slipping in the urine.

### Questions

1. What alternatives can you think of?

## Case 2

You are looking forward to meeting your new client, Mrs. Donald. However, when you arrive at her home, you encounter two large dogs. They are not going to let you in. Before you left home, you tried to call Mrs. Donald, however, she has no telephone.

### Questions

1. What do you do?
2. She cannot hear you and does not know what time you are coming. What choices do you have?

# Unit 9   Principles of Infection Control

## Case 1

You are caring for a teenage girl who has TB and is still contagious. When caring for her, you are required to use isolation precautions. However, she has several friends who are very uncooperative. Every time your back is turned, they are in her room. You have asked the parents for assistance. But as soon as they leave, the girls are back.

### Questions

1. What can you do?
2. How can you keep your client isolated?

## Case 2

Your client has measles. You have never had the measles.

### Questions

1. How would you care for your client without developing the measles?
2. What precautions would you use?

# Unit 10   From Wellness to Illness

## Case 1

You have been caring for Mrs. Moreno for several weeks. A nurse comes every week and sets up medications for the week. One of your responsibilities is to remind Mrs. Moreno to take her medication. When you arrive, you notice that she has not taken any medication all day. You remind her to take the medication. She tells you that God visited her and told her the medication is poisonous and not to take it. This is very unusual behavior for Mrs. Moreno.

### Questions

1. What would you do?
2. Who would you call?
3. How will you convince Mrs. Moreno to take her medication?

## Case 2

Your client, Mr. Pope is usually very talkative. Today, however, he seems very quiet. His voice seems a little slurred. His face droops on the right side. You take his vital signs and discover his blood pressure is 210/100. You know this is very dangerous.

### Questions

1. What do you do next?
2. How will you report his condition and at the same time keep him calm?

# Unit 11   Mental Health

## Case 1

You are caring for a client who is very depressed. Usually, she sits quietly looking out the window all day without talking. She will answer questions only with short answers. Today, when you arrive, Mrs. Jose is talking loudly, smiling, and seems very glad to see you.

### Questions

1. What do you think has happened?
2. Do you need to report this?

## Case 2

You are caring for Mr. Fife. He has a psychiatric diagnosis. He cannot care for his needs. You are to give him a bath, change his clothes, and prepare food for two meals. You are concerned about his careless smoking habits. He drops lighted matches on the floor. Sometimes, he will have as many as three cigarettes going at one time.

### Questions

1. What can you do to prevent a fire?
2. Do you need to report this behavior to anyone?
3. Is there someone who can advise you?

# Unit 12   Digestion and Nutrition

## Case 1

The client you are caring for is on a special diet. She is very fussy about her food. You have asked her to tell you what she would like to have you prepare for her lunch. You have prepared what she asked for. When you put the plate in front of her, she looks at you in disgust and states that you have not prepared what she asked for. You are very upset about this behavior. In fact, you are ready to grab your coat and leave.

### Questions

1. What other alternatives are there?
2. Can you think of another solution?
3. Can you think of any reason she would behave this way?

## Case 2

You are caring for Mr. Talimentes, who is very malnourished. His wife died several months ago. They were very close, and he has lost 30 pounds since she died. Your task is to prepare a high-calorie meal for him.

### Questions

1. What can you do to encourage him to eat?
2. Can you think of any way to make his food higher in calories?

# Unit 13  Elimination

## Case 1

You have been assigned to care for Mrs. Schultz. She has an indwelling catheter. You are to give her a bath, prepare a meal, and change the bed linens. After you have bathed her and prepared her meal, you assist her into a wheelchair to eat. When you return to clean up her dishes, you notice urine on the floor. You know she has a catheter in place.

### Questions

1. What would you check first?
2. What do you think is causing the leaking?
3. Do you need to notify anyone? If yes, who?

## Case 2

You are working with Mr. Pipo and part of your assignment included toilet training his bladder. You are to take him to the toilet every 2 hours. You have been doing this for more than a week. He seems to understand, but when you take him to the toilet, he cannot urinate. When you return him to bed, he urinates on the floor.

### Questions

1. What do you think is going on?
2. Do you think he is purposely not cooperating?
3. Can you talk to him about the problem?

# Unit 14  Integumentary System

## Case 1

Mrs. Rizzo has been your client for several months. She has had a stroke and is unable to turn in bed without your assistance. You have tried consistently to keep her off her back, but she will wiggle and squirm in the bed until she is back on her back. Today when you are bathing her, you notice broken skin on her coccyx.

### Questions

1. What do you do?
2. What can you tell her?
3. Who do you contact?
4. How do you care for the area with broken skin?

## Case 2

You have given your client a bath and dressed her in clean clothes. You go to the kitchen to prepare food. When you return, you find she has removed all of her clothing.

### Questions

1. What do you think caused her to do this?
2. What do you do?
3. How can you prevent this from happening again?

# Unit 15   Musculoskeletal System: Arthritis, Body Mechanics, and Restorative Care

## Case 1

Your client, Mrs. Iota, has severe arthritis. Part of your assignment is to perform range of motion exercise to her extremities. You also need to bathe her and straighten up her room.

### Questions

1. What time do you think would be the best time to perform these exercises?
2. Is there anything you can do to make these exercises less painful to Mrs. Iota?

## Case 2

You have been assigned a new client. Her name is Mrs. Pisa. You have been instructed to give her a bath and to help her into a wheelchair. When you arrive, you find Mrs. Pisa is bedbound and unable to assist with her care. She weighs in excess of 300 pounds. You will not be able to move her alone.

### Questions

1. What can you do?
2. Is there anyone who can help you?
3. How could this have been avoided?

# Unit 16   Nervous System

## Case 1

You have been assigned to a new client, Mr. Shoji. He is a 45-year-old man who has had his left lower leg amputated. Part of your assignment is to help attach the prosthesis and help him into the chair. When you are ready to help him, he tells you that he has never attached the prosthesis and expects that you will take care of it.

### Questions

1. What can you do?
2. How can you perform your assignment and not let him know that you have never done this before?
3. Can you think of anything you can say to him that will help?

## Case 2

You are assigned to Mrs. Suzy. You have not cared for her before, but you know from the case conferences that you attend each week that she is very particular about her care. You have been given directions to her home but are completely lost. You know she will be very upset when you arrive.

### Questions

1. What can you do?
2. What can you do to avoid this in the future?

# Unit 17  Circulatory System

## Case 1

Mrs. Jacinto has been assigned to you. She has recently had a heart attack. She is a very busy lady. She has several children and grandchildren. Part of her care includes rest, taking it easy, and no stress. She is having a difficult time complying with this. In fact, when you arrive, you find her in the kitchen cleaning.

### Questions

1. How are you going to help your client take it easy?
2. What can you tell her?
3. Can you think of any ways to help her get her needed rest?

## Case 2

Mr. Nature is on blood thinning medications. You have been instructed to watch for bleeding when you care for him. You notice that when he brushes his teeth, there is a small amount of bleeding in the sink.

### Questions

1. Do you think you need to contact the case manager?
2. Where else would you expect to see bleeding if he getting too many blood thinners?
3. Where would you find out?

# Unit 18  Respiratory System

## Case 1

You arrive at Mrs. Katz's home. You find her sitting on the couch. She is gasping for breath. You check her vital signs. Her temperature is 101°F, her pulse is 100 and thready, and her respirations are 30.

### Questions

1. What do you think is going on?
2. What do you need to do first?
3. Who would you contact?

## Case 2

When you arrive at Mrs. Kasper's home, you find that her family is giving her a birthday party. In the front room, Mrs. Kasper is sitting on the couch with her oxygen cannula in place. Her son is sitting next to her smoking. They have brought a large cake and are serving it with ice cream. You know Mrs. Kasper is on a very strict diet. She looks at you and you can tell she does not know how to handle this situation.

### Questions

1. What do you do first?
2. How will you handle the relatives without offending them?

# Unit 19  Reproductive System

## Case 1

You have been caring for Mrs. Phillips for several months. When you change her bed, you notice blood on the sheets. You ask her where the bleeding is coming from. She tells you that after all these years, she is having a period again. You know something is wrong. Mrs. Phillips is 85 years old.

### Questions

1. What would you tell her about the bleeding?
2. Who would you call?
3. What do you think is wrong?

## Case 2

Mr. Tomas has recently had a prostatectomy. You know that this surgery affects his ability to have sexual relations. He asks you when he will be able to have sex with his wife again.

### Questions

1. How will you answer him?
2. What can you tell him?
3. Who else do you need to inform about this situation?

# Unit 20   Endocrine System and Diabetes

## Case 1

You are caring for a new client, Mrs. Luau. She is diabetic and takes insulin every day. When you arrive, you ask her if she has taken her insulin. She informs you that she is out of insulin. She then asks you to purchase it for her. You tell her that you cannot purchase her insulin. She tells you that the other home health aides and nurses buy it for her. You know that she can afford to buy the insulin.

### Questions

1. What do you do?
2. How will she get her insulin?
3. Who will you call?

## Case 2

Mr. Lei is your new client. You have been assigned to bathe him and assist him in dressing. He takes a shower. When you are assisting him with his clothing, you notice that he has two rather large blisters on his left foot. When you ask him about them, he tells you not to worry about them because he gets them all the time. You know that he is diabetic and that wounds tend to be difficult to heal on diabetics.

### Questions

1. What do you do?
2. Who do you contact?
3. Do you need to do any special treatment to the blisters?
4. Is there anything you can do to prevent further injury to the blisters?

# Unit 21   Caring for the Client Who Is Terminally Ill

## Case 1

You are caring for a terminal client, Mr. Montes. He is having problems accepting the fact that he is terminal. He keeps telling you about the plans he is making for next summer. He has even offered to take you fishing to a special spot where he knows you will be able to catch a big fish.

### Questions

1. What stage of grieving is he in?
2. What can you do to help him accept the fact that he is dying?
3. How do you feel about working with him?

## Case 2

When you arrive at the home of your client, you find him alone. When you approach him you notice that he is very still. You feel his wrist for a pulse, and his hand is cold. You cannot find a pulse. You place your head close to his chest and you cannot hear any signs of breathing.

### Questions

1. What do you do first?
2. Do you need to call anyone? If so, who?

3. What about relatives?
4. You do not know whether he has any relatives nearby. How will you find out about this?

# Unit 22  Caring for the Client with Alzheimer's Disease

## Case 1

Your client is diagnosed with Alzheimer's disease. He is easily distracted, and you have had increasing problems is caring for him. When you are bathing him, he walks out of the shower and runs out the door. When you are helping him eat, he stands suddenly, knocking the food all over the floor.

### Questions

1. What can you do to modify these problems?
2. Is there any way to alter his behavior?

## Case 2

You have been working with Mr. Kai for several weeks. At a recent case conference, the team decided to try reminiscence with him.

### Questions

1. What will your role in this therapy be?
2. Describe reminiscence therapy?
3. Why is it successful with the elderly?

# Unit 23  Caring for the Client with Cancer

## Case 1

Your client, Mrs. Jonas, has been undergoing a course of chemotherapy. She has lost 20 pounds and is very thin. She is nauseated all the time. She feels very discouraged at times; she has told you that she thinks the chemotherapy will kill her before the cancer does.

### Questions

1. What can you do to improve her appetite?
2. Can you think of anything to tell her that will make her less discouraged?
3. Will these problems continue after her therapy is finished?

## Case 2

Your client, Mrs. Polaski, has recently been diagnosed with cancer. Her physician has explained the options to her. She has decided not to have chemotherapy or surgery. She has heard of an alternate cure for cancer. It involves taking up to 100 vitamin pills a day. You feel that the treatment she has chosen will not be successful.

### Questions

1. What do you do?
2. Will you be able to support her in her choice?
3. You know that she has the right to choose her treatment, but you are concerned that she has not chosen the correct treatment. How will you cope with your feelings?
4. Is there any other person you could contact?

# Unit 24   Caring for the Client with AIDS

## Case 1

You have been assigned to a client with AIDS. You have never cared for a seriously ill client before.

### Questions

1. What can you do to prepare yourself to care properly care for this client?
2. How do you feel about working with AIDS clients?
3. Does your client's life-style affect the way you care for him?
4. What would you do to make sure you give him excellent care?

## Case 2

Your client has AIDS. You are assigned to bathe him, do his laundry, and prepare his meals. The client lives with his family.

### Questions

1. What special care do you have to give to his clothes and bed linens?
2. Are there any special procedures that you need to follow in caring for his dishes?

# Unit 25   Maternal Care

## Case 1

Your client is 5 months pregnant. She is bleeding vaginally. This is her first pregnancy. She is emotionally distraught. You will need to care for her personal care needs and care for her household while she is on bed rest. You know that she is very upset.

### Questions

1. What can you do to help her cope with this problem?
2. What activities can she enjoy in bed?
3. Can you think of activities that you can participate in with her?

## Case 2

Your client has had a healthy baby girl. You have been hired to help her for a week so that she can get some extra rest before assuming the responsibilities of the entire household. The problem is her friends, who continually pop in to say hi. Your client does not want to tell them to leave.

### Questions

1. What can you do to help your client get her needed rest and not insult her friends?
2. Can you work out visiting times with her friends?

# Unit 26   Infant Care

## Case 1

You are caring for a client with a 6-week-old baby. You have been hired because the mother is at her wits end. The baby cries constantly. Mrs. Lopes cannot get any rest. She is emotionally unable to cope with the baby. She is convinced that the baby hates her.

### Questions

1. What can you do to help the baby ?
2. How can you comfort Mrs. Lopes?
3. What can you do to help Mrs. Lopes cope with the baby?

## Case 2

You are caring for Baby Maggie. Every time you feed her, she vomits. You have tried different formulas with the same result. Her mother is very concerned that you do not know how to feed babies.

### Questions

1. What do you think is happening?
2. How will you explain to the mother that something serious is wrong with the baby?
3. Should you contact your case manager?

# Unit 27   Job-Seeking Skills

## Case 1

You have completed your course as a home health aide. You applied for a position as a home health aide with Jones Home Health. You have been asked to come to an interview.

### Questions

1. How will you prepare for the interview?
2. What do you need to bring with you?
3. How will you dress for the interview?

## Case 2

You have arrived for your 11 AM interview. You are dressed appropriately. You have your certificates, your driver's license, your health statement, and other various papers. When you are called for your interview, the nurse who is conducting the interview states that you are an hour late. You check you daytimer, and sure enough, you were scheduled to be here 1 hour earlier.

### Questions

1. What do you do?
2. How can you let this nurse know that you are very interested in this job?
3. How can you prevent this from happening next time?